Insights to
Better
Living

Insights to Better Living

*Dive Into A Well-Being Lifestyle
With Lao Tzu*

by

Tham Trong Ma

INSIGHTS TO BETTER LIVING

Tham Trong Ma

Paperback ISBN: 978-1-954891-42-5
Ebook ISBN: 978-1-954891-41-8

CONTENTS

INTRODUCTION

The desires of man are insatiable such that when we create a goal and achieve it, we seek more, more money, influence, beauty, power, and the list goes on. It's no wonder the disharmony and imbalance we experience as individuals first, as a society, then as a nation, and lastly, the world at large. When we search deep within our hearts and critically get to the root of the violence and injustice we see in our environment, we can only come to one point, greed. Why do we seek more at the expense of others? Why is the Peace of our world threatened? Were we created for violence, famine, war, strife, and killings? Are natural disasters natural? Why does plastic surgery, feminism, racism, transgender, etc., seem to be the order of the day? These and many other questions have weighed the hearts of many of us.

In our search for happiness, freedom, wealth, and abundance, we forget that the things we seek must not conquer our inner Peace, Harmony, and Balance. The words Harmony, Balance, and Peace, if you notice, are repetitive. Peace is a state of tranquility, being free from thoughts and emotions that make you oppressed or restless. On the other hand, harmony is the ability to be united with yourself, being in togetherness with your personality, both good and evil, accepting your makeup. Finally, Balance is a state of equilibrium or stability. These highlighted words make up the foundation of Tao - The Way.

Earth, as we know it today, was not like this centuries ago. It was a scenic, picturesque, pleasant, and balanced place to live in. The energy (Qi) that flowed from its cardinal points brought Peace and abundance to humans and their inhabitants. What changed? The Earth or humans? The answer is quite glaring. We changed, and it affected the Earth's balance causing chaos and disrupting the flow of energy; hence, we experience natural (earthquakes, volcanic eruptions, hurricanes, etc.) and artificial disasters (global warming, desertification, oil spills, etc.).

The Way-Tao is a way of life that prioritizes Nature. Our oneness and balance with Nature will enlighten our spirits to see life's beauty and true essence. In this book, *"Insights To Better Living,"* we see a practical way to help us achieve the Harmony needed for our abundance while we journey through Earth.

As a famous quote goes, "where there is no law, there is no order." Laws, principles, codes of conduct, ethics, and punishments are put in place to govern our society effectively and put things in order. As humans, we have unique features that distinguish us from the other inhabitants of the Earth, such as; our components of higher, complex thinking, problem-solving skills, will, and expressive nature. Therefore, about The Book of Ethics by Lao Tzu, which talks about the Way and virtues that should govern our culture and belief systems in poems, this book was developed as a guide to help you reflect and live your life at its maximum potential.

That being said, the book is divided into three parts; Part 1- The Body, Part 2 - The Spirit, and Part 3 - The Harmony of the Body and Spirit. The body is the reason we exist on Earth. Without the body, there is no functioning, no life; in fact, all we hope to achieve will be shadows. Another quote says, "Health is Wealth." Honestly, it is indeed. We know individuals or even individuals with unharnessed potentials, strong drive, will, passion, great ideas, fantastic problem-solving skills, to mention a few but, we are limited for factors like age, environment, diet and nutrition, physical well-being. When we have a deteriorating body, we become hindrances to ourselves and also to others around us. Hence, the motivation for healthier living and hygiene. Taking care of your body is what you owe yourself to attain heights. You are responsible for what you eat and drink, and you also bear the consequences of the unhealthy lifestyle principles you live by. How do you perceive your body? How much worth have you accrued your body to be? Invest in your body, and it is the container that will get you before Kings and even make you one yourself.

Our spirit component is also vital in our quest for greatness and abundance. The state of our inner self and consciousness is discussed extensively in this book. Every mishap and violence happening in the world today was birthed from within. What is the state of your spirit? Have you learned to channel the flow of Nature's energy effectively? Why is our spirit essential? Out of the abundance of our hearts (spirit) yields the troubles of life. A lot of us do not pay attention to what or who we indeed are within. You can come to self-realization through meditation, yoga, and other healthy practices bolstered in the book.

Man is both body and spirit; both components are needed to be in Harmony with themselves. Harmony with our body components provides a balance that transcends to our environment, society, and our world at large. Every chapter of this book aims to spur us into a healthier and more natural way of living for our peace and world peace.

Going through every page and part of this book is an eye-opener that enlightens your spirit to live the right way. Never forget to be your number one motivation. You are the change the world needs. It has and will always begin with you. Be it and Earn it the Nature's Way.

Part I

THE BODY

Chapter One

THE ORIGIN OF THE
HUMAN BODY

In his book The Grand Design, physicist Stephen Hawking states that the laws of physics do not admit the possibility that the universe was created by God. If we reflect on the development of knowledge from the Renaissance to the present day, we can affirm that humanity is dismantling, relying on science, the entire set of religious beliefs about the world and nature, built or elaborated up to that historical moment. Modern science at the head of giants like Copernicus, Galileo, Kepler, Newton and closer to us, the entire generation of physicists at the beginning of the 20th century, has done nothing more than demonstrate that the universe is studied from itself, without need to resort to external forces. What Hawking does is reconfirm this current of thought.

The Catholic Church responded to these advances in the knowledge of nature with violence, burning alive (Giordano Bruno) or threatening to do so (Galileo), anyone who dared to disagree with its postulates of faith and its dogmatic beliefs. There is nothing so dangerous as the certainty of being in possession of the absolute truth. This belief has been the source of tragic human religious or political conflicts. Science, on the contrary, is not dogmatic, it proposes the openness and provisionality of knowledge.

This fact combines better with the flexibility present in the natural and social processes in which humans develop. The problem seems to be that unlike myth and religion which offer a vision of the whole and offer answers to all questions, science leaves a space of uncertainty since its answers are partial and feasible to reevaluate. With modernity, we then enter a world of true, verifiable but modifiable beliefs and we leave behind a world of false but coherent and total beliefs.

In any case, physics, despite its advances in the knowledge of the universe and the composition of matter, did not articulate with the human. The most forceful blow did not come then from this science, but from biology, from Darwin's theory about how species have evolved to give way to the many and wonderful diversity that is expressed before our eyes.

Darwin's theory thus becomes the greatest work of human thought by pointing out the mechanism by which all life on the planet has changed, has evolved in the course of time, how the offspring is modified from cumulative changes in time giving rise to some species giving rise to others, generating an ordered variability. Darwin, dismantled an idea fixed in the minds of men and reinforced by religious thought, the immutability of species. Men and women thought that species were fixed, that they did not change, that they had been created once and for all by a creator. Darwin proposed change, the mechanism

INSIGHTS TO BETTER LIVING

of natural selection that explains in a simple way, how some species can give rise to others. That is, we are all related. Marvelous!

Darwinian theory is completely sound and is accepted as fact today in the scientific community. There are discussions and debates but within the theory, not outside of it. It is a solid but open theory, not dogmatic. All the advances since the publication of Darwin's book have confirmed the fact of evolution. Paleontology and the fossil record, molecular biology and genome structure, comparative morphology, have offered empirical evidence about the evolutionary process.

Of course, religious ideas are part of our cultural heritage and are solid ideas in the minds of men, which permeate what we have been culturally. Religion and myth have helped us to endure the anguish generated by human consciousness. But religious ideas are only a possibility of our cognitive structure. The theory of evolution clashes head-on with the force of these ancient beliefs. But from 1543, the year of the publication of the book of Copernicus, the sun stopped rotating around the earth. And since 1859, the year of the publication of Darwin's book, the origin and diversity of species, including humans, ceased to have a creator. It is not easy to see and accept that there is no God, that we are simply one more species, like any other.

We should not fear seeing ourselves as is in the mirror. This blind and indifferent conception contains new ways of conceiving our lives. If we are able to recognize ourselves as a species, that therefore we are genomically related to distant and close species in the phylogeny, that we come from the natural world, whether we want to or not, we make a unity with that world, then a new ethic based in respect for nature so necessary in the face of predation practiced by current societies.

On the other hand, the idea of the absence of a creator, of a protective father, of a superior being to whom we can turn in moments of anxiety and anguish, generates psychological and corporeal distress. Thinking like this leads to a feeling of infinite loneliness. But that is precisely the human side of evolutionary theory. We are not dependent on anyone except ourselves. The course of humanity will be the sole responsibility of humanity itself. We are products of our own decisions. Like any species, we live on the edge, always on the edge, but extinction or survival will be the result of our own actions.

This awareness of loneliness, of who we really are, should lead us to recognize the value of human relationships. Perhaps we are alone as a species, but not as individuals, since we count on others as support and traveling companions. That should be enough for us.

- **Scientific perspectives**
  The field of human evolution constitutes a multidisciplinary field of research, Paleoanthropology, highly controversial and in a constant state of boiling and change. In fact, the world related to our origins has revealed remarkable complexity and generated heated debates from the very moment that the theory of evolution was accepted by the scientific community.

Australopithecus afarensis

The subject is prone to multiple disagreements because it is an aspect of biological thought with a tendency to subjectivity, something that, on the other hand, is recognized today in practically all scientific work. But in addition, the interpretation of human origins has been overloaded with considerable gender bias. Let us clarify that with the term "gender" we refer not only to the biological differences between one sex and the other of the human species, but also to the social and cultural differences attributed to people based on their sex.

It is revealing to bear in mind that Paleanthropology is a recently created scientific discipline (early 20th century) and, practically until the 1970s, the vast majority of scholars dedicated to the subject were men. This situation has caused the interpretation of our evolutionary history to have been polarized by a notable androcentrism, that is, the identification of the masculine with the human in general. In this context, and despite the great variation in explanatory models proposed over the years, there has been a common denominator: giving the female sex a very insignificant role in such a significant process.

Homo Sapiens

Until just a few decades ago, scholars viewed women as simply passive participants in evolutionary change, and limited themselves to relegating them to the role of giving birth, feeding, and caring for their young. While, on the contrary, men were described as responsible for many of the innovations that define us as humans, for example, the emergence of bipedal gait, brain enlargement, tool-making, cooperative communication or symbolic representation.

Thus, it should not be surprising that research related to our evolution has, and still does, carry away the conventional sexist bias that has permeated the academic world and the models it produces for centuries. In reality, evolutionary studies have not moved in a vacuum, but immersed within the same line as the cultural history of the West. In fact, we all carry a "baggage": our gender matters, just as it matters who our teachers were, where we study, when we study, what our religion is, our cultural heritage, and so on. As the American biologist Ruth Hubbard has noted, among others: "There is no such thing: an objective, value-free science."

It can therefore be said that the androcentric bias that has weighed down studies on human evolution has been present since Darwin placed humanity within the evolutionary framework.

The recognized and admired father of the theory of evolution, following a tradition that came from ancient times, admitted without qualms, at least publicly, the superiority of man over woman as an indisputable characteristic of nature. We find it interesting to highlight the deep sexism that permeated Darwinian thought, one of the most influential in the history of biology.

Darwin's theory left women in the gutter of evolution
The Darwinian revolution, which changed so many things and swept away so many prejudices from the natural sciences, did not change the view held for centuries about the "natural" inferiority of women with respect to men. The only notable change in this regard was that hierarchical differences between

the human sexes, previously attributed to the god or gods, were now attributed to science.

Although many have blamed the English naturalist for the evolutionary underestimation of the female sex, many experts today claim that it was mainly some of his exalted followers - "more Darwinists than Darwin" - who defended such marginalization most emphatically.

However, The Origin of Man, the book in which Darwin devoted more space to women, was a clear reflection of its author's attempt to turn this ancient prejudice into "scientific truth": women "by nature" are inferior to men. The scientist affirmed that many of the typical faculties of the female sex (intuition, rapid perception and perhaps also those of imitation) "are proper and characteristic of inferior races, and therefore correspond to a past and lower state of culture."

In contrast to these feminine characteristics, she emphasized that "the man developed superior mental faculties, such as observation, reason, invention or imagination" that, finally, made him superior to women in all areas. Darwin concluded: "in body and spirit man is more powerful than woman."

To explain male supremacy, the famous Briton, and most of his innumerable followers, resorted to the different functions that the two sexes of the human species fulfilled. Since the natural function of men was to support and protect women and their young, they had to fight for survival in dangerous activities that required great intelligence. This obligation of care and supply was the engine that led them to develop great courage, aggressiveness and energy.

Nature, on the other hand, made less demands on women since, being their only activity procreation and nurturing, their role was purely physical. They hardly fought, their food supply to the group was secondary, they did not have to solve new situations or face risks, challenges, etc. The reproduction and care of the offspring required only passive and domestic maternal qualities.

Supported by this reasoning, Darwin argued that the value of a woman lay in her reproductive organs. And, since neither the development of a child in the womb, nor delivery or milk production depended on the female ability to think, they did not require that their brains and minds evolve at a speed equal to that of males.

Male activity
Darwinian reasoning further held that men in general had acquired the ability to think first; as this trait was crucial for survival it then passed to women, which allowed them to evolve as well. In other words, thanks to the fact that girls and boys inherit the characters in an equivalent way, the evolution ran evenly for both sexes. In this sense, the naturalist reflected: "if it were not for the law of equality in the transmission of inheritance, the physical and intellectual difference that separates us from women would still be greater than it is."

Only when referring to reproduction, in Chapter IV of The Origin of Man, Darwin attributed to women an important evolutionary role. According to the scientist, in most species the members of one sex, usually the male, compete with each other for access to mating with the other sex. But, he also considered that female predilections for accepting a mate had an influence: the chosen males achieved greater reproductive success compared to those who were not chosen.

In this regard, he wrote: «In courtship, of the two sexes, the male is the most active member. The female, on the other hand, with very rare exceptions, is less impatient than the male… she [although] shy and passive, in general exercises some choice and accepts a male preferring him over others.

It is evident that the core of the Darwinian thesis contained a contradiction: the female sex carries out the sexual choice but at the same time its attitude is one of great passivity. This is a paradox that was hardly discussed when the book came out. Rather to the contrary, it was overlooked. In fact, efforts were concentrated on underlining the subordinate role in which the great scientist had placed women.

Finally, it is interesting to insist that The Origin of Man (1871) generated an avalanche of discussions and endless replies among the scientific community and in society in general, both at the time it was published and later.

However, with regard to the situation of women, saving the last decades, there have been almost no controversies that reached the general public, but rather a tacit majority acceptance of Darwinian theses. In reality, it should not surprise us too much since these theses hardly changed the dominant conceptions and no one felt, at least openly, offended or surprised by the sexist content of the work of such a famous author.

Today, although considerably less widespread than in the past, androcentrism still persists. And this is not a marginal abnormality. As the American essayist Adrienne Rich has so well pointed out: "objectivity is the name given in patriarchal society to male subjectivity."

- **Religious perspectives**
  The religious perspective about the origin of man is the belief of a divine creation is responsible for the life and the universe, contrary to scientific consensus that supports a natural means of evolution.

Since evolutionary phenomena have been described in astronomy, geology and biology, creationists (those who believe in religious part of human origin) have maintained controversy in this regard, because the scientific explanation of these phenomena is not compatible with their interpretation of religious texts. The debate raises important political issues, in particular in matters of education, scientific research, freedom of opinion and beliefs.

Creationist currents show a great diversity, from those who support fixism by developing a theory of theistic nature ("Jeune-Terre creationism" and "Vieille-Terre") to those with more deistic positions who embrace the transformist theory (hypothesis of the intelligent design and directed panspermia).

The "Creationism Young-Earth reads the Bible or the Koran as scientific and historical books, conveying the belief that the story of the creation of the universe, as provided by religious texts, gives a literally accurate description of origin of the

Universe. This literal interpretation of texts like Genesis is based on the conviction that these texts were "dictated by God" as absolute, definitive and indisputable truths (the case of certain Protestant churches, the majority in the Bible Belt of the United States). This current of thought is generally associated with the rejection of any idea of biological and geological evolution.

Most monotheistic religious traditions (Judaism, Christianity and Islam) postulate the creation of the world by a supreme God. The fundamentalist reading is refused by the majority of current Christian Churches, which favor a hermeneutical reading.

For Catholics, the creation of the universe by God is not in itself opposed to evolution: creation is above all the relationship between creatures and a Creator, their first principle.

Creationism is not, however, restricted to currents that interpret religious texts literally, but also includes Old-Earth creationism which admits that the universe is well over 6000 years; the partisans of intelligent design, of currents which admit aspects of the theory of evolution but exclude man from it; theistic evolution which admits that the evolution of species takes place but that it is directed or influenced by divinities or a Creator who would give birth to the universe, to the living and to the mechanisms allowing them then to evolve by them.

According to creationism, everything starts from God. The stance of creationism suggests certain philosophical dilemmas: How did the world came to be? Is it even possible to create something from nothing?

There is a metaphysical principle that "nothing comes out of nowhere." If the universe, which encompasses everything that exists, had an origin, it would have arisen out of nowhere, nullifying the aforementioned principle. To overcome this contradiction, it would be necessary to accept that the universe always existed. For creationism, that existence is given by God, who is eternal and has always existed.

As aforesaid, creationism is often claimed to be opposed to the theory of evolution proposed by Charles Darwin. This scientist explained that species, including humans, are derived from others. This would therefore assume that God did not create man out of nothing. For creationists, on the other hand, each species is the fruit of an act of divine creation.

A part of the Christian creationists assure that our planet is young, so young that it does not reach 10,000 years old; more specifically, they usually point out that it was created by the god Yahweh 6000 years ago, as described in the Ussher-Lightfoot Calendar. In other words, this ideology does not take into account scientifically based theories of the emergence of the universe and the Earth.

Many Protestant churches in North America support the Young Earth vision: Statistically, this is the theory that is respected by approximately 47% of North Americans, and about 10% of Christian universities teach it in their classrooms. Some Christian organizations, such as the Creation Research Institute and the Creation Research Society, also believe in this ideology.

To find the age of our planet mentioned above, which does not exceed six thousand years, the followers of this branch of creationism rely on deductions and calculations based on the ages of the characters in the Bible, as mentioned in Genesis and Other books. Young Earth creationism is divided into three views:

- The one that rejects the theory of the evolution of species categorically, as well as any indication of evolution of planet Earth, according to geological studies. This is the most common form of ideology;
- The one that is subtitled "ambiguous", which contemplates the possibility that all living beings except human beings have evolved;
- The so-called "of a rapid evolution", according to which the god Yahweh carried out the creation in a few days, so that the evolution did take place but it occurred in just one week.

In the field of literature, finally, creationism is the name of a poetic movement that emerged in the early twentieth century, postulating the absolute autonomy of the poem. According to this movement, the poem does not reflect the appearance of nature, but rather follows its internal logic and impulses.

Chapter Two

THE UNION OF THE HUMAN BODY AND MIND

Life is a matrix - the ancient Greek thinker Plato, made this idea clear in the allegory of the cave: There are people chained in a cave and only see images of the real world - as shadows that a fire casts into the cave from outside. What we perceive with our senses is only a flawed copy of a perfect world that exists independently of space and time. A sphere is round, this truth always applies, regardless of whether all seemingly round objects have dents and corners under the microscope.

Reality is thus divided into two parts ("dualism"): into an eternally immaterial "world of ideas" and a physically perishable "world of senses". While the latter can deceive us as in the allegory of the cave, infallible knowledge lies in the world of ideas, where the idea of a sphere or of the "beautiful in itself" exists objectively. We only get there from the cave through our thinking - because our spirit lives in the immortal soul, which is temporarily trapped in the body, but actually comes from the world of ideas. If we use our reason, the soul can remember the ideas and thus also recognize what is good and just. But the body also plays a central role in Plato's educational ideal.

Through sport, we learn to control our body with its desires and thus also train our soul. But the body also plays a central role in Plato's educational ideal.

- **According to Aristotle, there is no thinking without a body;**
  Aristotle wants to turn the philosophy of his teacher Plato upside down on its feet. For him, the essence of things is not in the ideas, but in the things themselves. Without the football and all the apparently round objects, we would not come up with the idea of rounding things off. So the idea reflects what the senses perceive.
  With this, Aristotle rehabilitates sensory perception - and introduces an immortal soul through the back door. For Aristotle, as for Plato, this is a universal principle that breathes life into the body, but is itself immaterial. A part of the soul, the "active spirit", is even immortal - if only as a kind of cosmic principle that breaks free from every individuality after human death. Because here Aristotle is again a materialist - and empiricist: thoughts are only filled with content through perception.

- **You can think without a body, Descartes believes;**
  The French René Descartes was a notorious skeptic. Because not only the senses deceive us, but also our intellect, for example when we dream, Descartes questioned everything. What remained was the doubt - and the thinking: "I think, therefore I am." So thinking is also possible without a

body, because the world breaks down into two independent substances: the soul as the immaterial inner world of free thinking ("res cogitans") As well as the physical ("res extensa"), which as pure matter follows natural laws.

Contrary to ancient beliefs, however, the soul does not need it for life. Perception and movement are mechanical - with which (unreasonable) animals become "machines". But the human being is a double being with body and immortal soul.   The aim is to give the reasonable mind control over the weak body. But how do mind and body actually interact? Because Descartes asked himself this question, he is considered the father of the "body-soul problem" - which he was only able to solve in an unsatisfactory manner. To substantiate the mutual influence of body and mind, he claimed that the soul sits in the middle of the brain in the pineal gland.

- **For Marx, property and power relations shape our ideals;** For the famous critic of capitalism Karl Marx, thinking depends on the economy. "It is not the consciousness of people that determines their being, but their social being that determines their consciousness." In "dialectical materialism" being and consciousness are indeed in a kind of interaction, but ultimately social and individual beliefs depend above all on it economic, historical and social conditions.

Ownership and power relations thus significantly shape our ideals of beauty as well as ideas of justice or freedom. Because in capitalism, this often serves to maintain power structures instead of the well-being of the people, Marx also speaks of "false consciousness". But the world is not determined: a change in conditions is possible.

- **There is agreement that the body has influence over the mind;**
  In 1979, the American neurophysiologist Benjamin Libet caused a sensation with an experiment. Subjects should raise their hands at a freely chosen time. The measurement of the brain activity showed that the unconscious neural impulse to move was present before the conscious decision.

Are the human mind and consciousness materialistically reducible to nerve activities? This would reduce our free will and also the jurisprudence based on the question of guilt is absurdum.

Other scientists are more cautious because the experiment has a weak point: the test subjects already knew what action to take, and an active decision was no longer necessary.

In another experiment recently, the researcher John-Dylan Haynes showed that that our consciousness can affect unconscious decisions. In any case, the debate continues to this day, especially philosophers disagree with neuroscientists.

They doubt that complex rational decisions can be explained in the same way as simply raising one's arm. What the brain researchers remind us in any case is the influence of the body on our mind.

- **The body is punished and trimmed by the powerful, says Foucault;**
  The French philosopher Michel Foucault sees the body determined by social power structures - and disciplined by those in power. The Church preaches abstinence and fidelity and makes human sexuality the subject of religious laws and discussions.

  In the Middle Ages and under absolutism, confessions were extracted under torture and physical torture was a widespread punishment. The destruction of the body of a delinquent was also a popular discipline. In the 18th and 19th centuries, the obvious brutality increasingly faded from discipline, and according to Foucault, the body is now made more subtle in public institutions, in prisons, but also in schools, orphanages, clinics and in the military.

  In this way, power structures are internalized by the individual. The aim is, as it were, their submission and the increase in economic usefulness. "The human body enters a machine of power that penetrates, dissects and reassembles it. [...] In this way, the discipline fabricates subjugated and trained bodies, docile and passive bodies." For Foucault, the body is the surface on which power is inscribed.

- **Spivak sees the female body as exploited in capitalism;**
  For Gayatri Spivak, a co-founder of the post-colonial theory, who sees the current balance of power as a continuation of colonial structures of rule and strives to overcome them, the female body in countries in the global south is the scene of patriarchal supremacy and sufferers of global inequality.

Transnational corporations realize their profits on the backs of the workers in the low-wage countries. In the context of unrestrained capitalism, women become objects of exploitation, without the possibility of political participation or self-representation - because, if at all, others are talking about them.

According to Spivak, this is also to be understood as a criticism of the hegemonic tradition of many supposed liberation discourses by Western intellectuals.

- **Butler believes that the body and mind are subject to cultural norms;**
  According to contemporary philosopher Judith Butler, physical reality is also shaped by how we talk about something. As soon as the midwife says: "This is a boy", many allegedly follow typical male attributions. As early as the 1970s, feminists took up the distinction between biological (sex) and social sex (gender), which came from psychoanalysis and sociology, to point out the oppression of women and the fact that gender roles are socially constructed.

  Butler, being a feminist, rejects the Descartes-related dualism between supposedly unchangeable nature (sex) and culture (gender) - ultimately between body and mind. This maintains the separation between "man" and "woman" and the associated power relations.

- **Ending the debate about body and mind interaction;**
  This has always been a problem that keeps human beings arguing all the time. That is: Does the body control the mind or the mind control the body? The philosophers participating

in the debate have their own opinions, which can be roughly divided into two viewpoints: materialism and idealism.

The mind and body are not two incompatible aspects. Both the mind and the body are part of our life, and both are expressions of life. We should understand their relationship on the basis of seeing life as a whole.

Foreseeing one's own actions in advance is the most critical role of the soul. Knowing this, we can realize: how the mind controls the body - the mind sets the direction of the next action for the body.

If we don't have a direction to work hard, but only receive some scattered movement signals, it is useless. Since the mind can determine the direction of our actions, it occupies a pivotal position in life. At the same time, the mind is also affected by the body, the body is the executor of the action, and the mind can only exercise commanding powers within the scope of the body's abilities. For example, if the mind wants the body to run to the moon in the sky, it is nonsense unless it can overcome the limitations of the human body.

The horse and the horse rider are a vivid metaphor. The horse rider can direct the horse to go, but he cannot specify the details precisely. It cannot be forced. It can only be guided. In the end, it will be decided by the horse.

Mankind's ability to foresee the future will definitely develop in the long term, and mankind will work hard for the goals set by itself in order to consolidate the important position of mankind in the environment.

By studying the meaning contained in the various expressions of the individual, find a suitable way to understand the object, and compare his goals with the goals of other people.

In most cases, the mind affects the body. When a person thinks about something in his head, he will work hard on the matter, and finally give feedback to the body.

Chapter Three

THE COMPONENTS OF
THE HUMAN BODY

Endowed with gesture and speech, the human body is distinguished from that of animals by a whole series of physical characteristics, the inventory of which has undoubtedly not finished being drawn up: true bipedalism, liberation of the hand, capacity cranial.

Whether the differences are accentuated or blurred depending on the animal species to which he is compared, he nonetheless remains a singular being, and requires, as such, a specific approach. Inert or alive, all other bodies appear as objects placed in space, partes extra partes, in an exteriority and a distance conducive to cognitive reflection.

The human body, as composed of flesh and bones, can certainly be analyzed as a being in itself, but this mode of apprehension ignores its particularity and its incomparable character to other bodies. To truly understand him and to grasp something other than his remains, you have to change people and go from the third to the first.

So then, what are the components that makes up the body?

- **The brain: The seat of desires and emotions**
  The brain is made up of three major parts: the neocortex, the limbic system, and the reptilian system. The latter represents the primary brain, responsible for instincts (survival, flight...). The limbic system is the center of emotions and memory. The neocortex represents the center of higher cognitive functions and thus concerns, for example, strategy, spatial and long-term reasoning, perception, conscious thought or even language. The latter, the neocortex or "new brain", developed from the limbic system in the evolutionary history of the human brain, which could explain the crucial role of emotions on the functioning of the brain and especially of thought.

Until a few years ago, the location of emotions in the brain was localized by the scientific community exclusively to the limbic system. It was established that emotions run a single systematic genetic circuit. But advances in research have made it possible to discover that the areas of the brain causing emotion are multiple. As the neuropsychologist Aroa Gomez Marin tells us: "We know that the different emotions are not the result of the activation of a single cerebral structure: but that they are the result of the activation of a circuit of determined connections that allow communication between different areas of the brain."

Other theories agree on this point: the areas affected by emotions in our brain are numerous. They further argue that there would be no genetically established circuits in our brains.

The circuits responsible for the appearance of emotions would, on the contrary, be the result exclusively of the learning process: through our experiences or through language.

In terms of functioning, there is an important emotional circuit to know in order to understand the power of emotions in our brain. Joseph LeDoux, American neurologist, was the first to show the central role of the amygdala in the emotional circuit of our brain. This small organ explains that man is able to act following an emotion even before his thought system has been able to make a decision. "Anatomically, the system that governs emotions can act independently of the neocortex. Certain reactions and certain emotional memories can be formed without the slightest intervention of consciousness, of cognition," describes Joseph LeDoux.

When the brain receives sensory signals, two pathways are taken in parallel by the information received. Take the example of an emotional reaction of fear following a visual signal: that of the appearance of a tarantula in our field of vision (do you feel the shiver run through your arms and your back at this thought?). Let's get back to how our brains work:

The visual signal leaves the retina during the vision of this tarantula to go to the thalamus.

The thalamus is then responsible for transmitting information, according to the language of our brain, to the visual cortex.

The visual cortex is ultimately responsible for analyzing the received signal to find the necessary response.

If the appropriate solution is of an emotional nature, the signal will again be transmitted from the neocortex to the amygdala, located in the limbic system and therefore at the center of emotional controls.

But in parallel with this path, part of the signal is sent by a single synapse, by the thalamus directly to the amygdala, and can thus generate an emotional response very quickly. This fast track nevertheless remains primitive and detached from any cognitive analysis. It is thus completed a posteriori by the path taken by the neocortex, which can establish a more elaborate and adequate plan of action.

Emotions can thus be triggered without the slightest intervention of thought and gain the upper hand over reason for a given time, before the cognitive system has been able to analyze the information rationally. If this operation has saved lives many times in human history, it can also be the source of an inappropriate reaction in our daily lives.

The role of the amygdala in emotional memory should not be overlooked. This instance of our modus operandi is an essential guide in our choices. Indeed, Antonio Damasio has studied the role of the amygdala in decision making. He studied personal or professional choices, small or very important. His studies have shown that emotions and feelings are essential when making rational decisions. They are warnings to guide our choices in the right direction, the one where reason can be best used thanks to the emotional memory stored throughout our life.

Two forms of intelligence, therefore, inhabit our mind, our brain: intellectual intelligence and emotional intelligence. Intellectual intelligence has long been considered the only intelligence, but as Antonio Damasio says: after the paradigm of intellectual intelligence, the new objective is to link reason and emotions to better decide!

- **The blood: The familial bond**
  The natural bond of parents with their children and also that of the latter between them has always been considered "blood". It has the psychological value of an identity affinity of ways of being, the confirmation of which is sought in the physical and character similarity. The natural bond, of which we now know the genetic constitution, is the foundation of a relationship that is claimed to be defined from the start, in its own right.

In reality, the particularity of the bond between parents and children and between siblings is built, for better or for worse, through their relationships never detached from the environment outside the family.

The difference in the parents' relationship with their adopted children compared to that with their natural children can be significant only for the more complicated mutual investment, which there can be, certainly not for irrelevant biological reasons. The blood bond is a relatively recognized belief that supports the defensive and misleading need to separate the value of family relationships from their actual erotic/affective quality.

The only blood bond that has a relational meaning corresponds to the fact that we meet the world for the first time through close contact with the maternal body, after having lodged within it. The blood of this body fed us. By virtue of this exceptional common psychocorporeal experience, the mother invests us in an exceptional way as soon as we are born (and waiting for this to happen). A special recognition to which we respond in an equally special way.

The blood bond with the mother, to which Jewish law associates the right of citizenship, would lead to our annexation to a maternal universe closed to otherness and entertaining a "hit and run" relationship with the world, if it were not animated from the law of desire, the law of equal differences of desiring subjects. The equality of differences requires the structuring presence of the erotic relationship between the parents which assigns a function of equalizing redistribution of the currents of desire within the family to the father: the one who does not come from the womb of the mother and does not have a blood bond with her nor with the children.

The responsibility of parents towards their children that gives them greater blame if they harm them. This does not change in anything due to the fact that they have adopted them instead of procreating them. They are committed to taking good care of them because they are human beings whose destiny is heavily dependent on their dedication. This care, which they can be called to account for, will not bring it to fruition because it is part of their natural prerogative, which does not really bind them, but because they are capable of loving while respecting the particularity of the loved object. On this level, each child is adopted: he is not treated by his parents as his own extension, but is recognized and accepted in his difference and loved by taking care of it.

The law of blood contradicts the principle of universal brotherhood which ignores natural bonds and is based on the equal exchange between our different declinations of the common human matter. It violates the foundation of justice, it is an unjust law.

- **The limbs: Tools for creation**

    "The hand is the man himself." - *Anaxagoras*
    Anaxagoras affirms that man is the most intelligent of animals thanks to having hands; so it is reasonable to say that he got the hands because he is the smartest.

Hands are in fact an instrument, and nature, as an intelligent person would do, always attributes each of them to those who can use them; since it is more convenient to give flutes to someone who is already a flutist than to attribute the art of the flute to someone who owns flutes.

Nature attributes the lesser to the greater and more important, not the noblest and the greater to the lesser. So if this is the best way, and nature in the field of possibilities realizes the best one, then it is not that man is the most intelligent thanks to his hands, but he has hands thanks to being the most intelligent of animals.

Simply put, the most intelligent must be the one who properly knows how to use the greatest number of tools; now the hand seems to constitute not one but several instruments: in a certain sense it is an instrument in charge of other instruments.

Therefore, to him who is able to master the greatest number of techniques, nature has given, with his hand, the instrument capable of using the greatest number of other instruments.

As for those who maintain that man is not well constituted, indeed worse than all other animals (they say in fact that he has no protection for his feet, he is naked and without combat weapons), their speech is incorrect. The other animals have only one means of defense, and they are not allowed to replace it with another, on the contrary they must sleep and do anything else while always keeping, so to speak, their shoes on their feet, that is, without putting down the armor they have on their body nor can they change the weapon that has befallen them.

Man, on the other hand, is granted many means of defense, and he can always change them, also adopting the weapon he wants and when he wants it. In fact, the hand can become a claw, hoof, horn, or even a spear, sword and any other weapon or tool: all this can be because everything can grasp and hold.

The shape of the hand was also designed by nature in this sense. It can be articulated and divided into several parts, because the capacity for cohesion is also implicit in the division, while the first is not implicit in the second. And it is possible to use it as a single organ, two or many.

Aristotle has this to say in his book – "The Parts of Animals"

"It is not because he has hands that man is the most intelligent of beings, but because he is the most intelligent of beings that he has hands. Indeed, the most intelligent being is the one who is able to use the greatest number of tools well: the hand does indeed seem to be not one tool, but several. Because it is, so to speak, a tool that takes the place of others. It is therefore to the being capable of acquiring the greatest number of techniques that nature has given by far the most useful tool, the hand.

Also those who say that man is not well constituted and that he is the least well shared among animals (because they say he is without shoes, he is naked and has no weapons to fight) are in error. Because the other animals each have only one means of defense and it is not possible for them to change it for another, but they are forced, so to speak, to keep their shoes on to sleep and to do anything, what else, and should never put down the armor they have around their body or change the weapon they have been shared. Man, on the contrary, has many means of defense, and he is always free to change them and even have the weapon he wants when he wants. For the hand becomes a claw, hoof, horn or lance or sword or any other weapon or tool. She can be all of that, because she is able to grab everything and hold everything."

Intelligence is the faculty of inventing means to achieve an end. Suffice to say that his approach is always to manufacture tools. The invention, the manufacture, the use of tools are therefore all elements of the first approach specific to intelligence. For Aristotle, nature is wise: it would be foolish to give a tool to someone who does not have the intelligence to use it. To man, because he is the most intelligent being in nature, nature has given an organ which he is able to use: the hand, not as a tool, but as a multiplicity of tools.

Modern anthropology proves Aristotle and his finalism wrong. But the image of the hand, the tool of tools, remains beautiful and strong.

- **The tongue: The vehicle for propagating ideas**
  The tongue is one of the essential members of the human body. It is precisely because of the existence of the tongue that we can taste the taste of various foods and know what is sour, what is sweet, what is bitter, and what is spicy. Therefore, for the tongue, the most important role is to be able to sense taste. Of course, our human tongue also has other functions, which can be specifically manifested in the following aspect; speaking.

The role of auxiliary speaking
We should all know that human beings cannot only speak without their vocal cords, but also an important organ, the tongue. The tongue is a heavy-duty organ that assists in pronunciation. Without the tongue, we humans cannot speak or pronounce at all.

Human have the vital need to relate. These relationships in the social context are possible thanks to communication, which implies entering into relationships with others and an exchange of views, since we are alternately emitters and receivers.

Communicating is, then, expressing or manifesting to others our thoughts, desires and our interpretations of things and the world. All this, however, is not possible without language, since it is through it that communication relationships are established.

Now, what then is language? Well, in a broad and even metaphorical sense, people often speak of the "language" of flowers, stars, hills, and so on. Animals that live in a community also have very subtle communication procedures, as in the case of bees and ants. However, all this is not language in the strict sense.

Language becomes a unique and exclusively human activity, which allows us to communicate and relate to our fellow human beings through the expression and understanding of messages. In other words, language is the ability that everyone has to communicate with others using oral, written or other signs.

This concept of language, as it can be understood, has a broader significance than the production of articulated sounds that make up words and phrases.

a. There is language through symbols such as traffic signs, military signs, etc.
b. There is body language such as mimicry and gestures.
c. There is language expressed through linguistic codes, which is the most important means of human communication, which is called oral language or speech.

It is this latter form of language that is addressed in this book. It becomes a personal act in which the speaker emits a message using the signs and rules that he needs at a given moment.

Language, then, is a very important quality of the human being thanks to which it communicates, knows its past, can analyze, interpret and understand its present and, consequently, project itself into the future as an individual and as a social being.

Why is speaking important?
To highlight its importance, it should be noted first of all that human beings live immersed in a veritable verbal ocean, in a world or an eminently competitive social reality, where the word, especially that expressed verbally, is a decisive factor that constitutes the bridge, the noose, the weapon, the important means or instrument of union or disunity; of understanding or misunderstanding; of success, recognition or indifference; of failure, frustration or marginalization among human beings. In other words, speech becomes a vital process that enables communication with others, increasing the opportunity to live better in a society like the current one.

Thus, all human beings need verbal language to express our needs, thoughts, feelings and emotions; We even need it to solve the most basic things in our life: hunger, thirst, shelter, work. We also need it to acquire knowledge, to abstract and project ourselves symbolically and truly in time and space, as well as to communicate and adapt to the environment.

We can do all this thanks to verbal language; But when there are defects in this quality, a series of problems are generated that can limit and marginalize us socially.

Having said that, it is important to understand that the tongue is an essential instrumental aspect for the life of relationship. Without it, man is a socially mutilated being, without the ability to project himself symbolically. It is also considered as a fundamental aspect for the development of intelligence and for all cognitive activity related to life. However, it is good to point out that this quality does not refer to a purely "mechanical" fact, nor to something that is acquired or given in a natural way, such as learning to walk, but rather it is something much more complex, and that behind of all this is the fact of feeling and thinking well, having a personality and being a man.

The child and the power of language
Since birth, the child lives in an eminently verbal context, where people, radio, television and a thousand and one other forms of interrelation establish verbal bridges with him; that is, the child at birth passes from the "amniotic bath" of the mother's womb to the "verbal bath" of the social environment, which becomes the conditioning factor for the acquisition and development of language.

This social environment with its manifestations of language, not only surrounds the child but also makes him or her receive and assimilate it directly, since the child is spoken to from the first day of birth together with the physical demonstrations of affection: hugs, kisses, caresses and tender words almost sung.

This influence of the sociolinguistic environment makes the child, at first, associate verbalizations with situations of human contact and feelings of well-being, constituting a strong incentive for the acquisition of language. Later, as you progress, you become aware of its instrumental value for the demands and requests related to your needs.

The child, around the eighth month of birth, discovers that certain types of vocalizations manage to attract adults around him (call function), which begins to explode. In this we can see the beginning of a vocal communication relationship that later became the core of all verbal activity.

In the second year of life, the child discovers the power of the word, particularly the "name." He realizes that just by naming objects or actions adults obey him, either by bringing the objects closer to him or by performing the actions. In addition, he also obtains verbal answers on the topic he proposes, which is enriching and facilitating his linguistic development. Later the child will use this quality as a means of "controlling" and "directing" the actions of others and, later, of himself.

Thus, at different stages of acquisition there are different motivations to keep going. However, the deep roots of these motivations must be traced in affective relationships within the family, since without this support language either does not develop to its full potential, or it atrophies. Hence, the affective family climate and the opportunities provided by parents for the child to practice language are basic conditions for the establishment, development or subsistence of this quality.

Thus, thanks to tongue, the child is overcoming the here and now; You can draw on knowledge from experience to solve current problems and plan for the future.

The tongue also enables you to interact more fully with other people and share your individual world of fantasies, beliefs, hopes, and regrets.

In this way, human beings have been using the tongue to create huge and complex civilizations, and they continue to use it to promote scientific and technological progress. Unquestionably, language, speech, is one of the instruments of enormous importance and power.

The language and the psychological adjustment of the child
When the acquisition of speech is done within an environment of security, love and understanding; When this learning takes place in a family environment without tension, with mature and happy parents, all obstacles are simple and easily overcome by the child, reaching the different stages of development in an expected period that may vary, but with a certain graduation in that acquisition.

Thus, children who come from balanced homes, in which their parents provide them with love, security, stimulation and understanding, are generally happy children who express themselves normally, confident of themselves and with a wide disposition for relationships with others, the rest. This also means that they have the best possibilities to develop harmonically and integrally, adapting adequately to their sociolinguistic environment.

Instead, let's imagine the origin of those children or young people who feel disabled or affected in this quality that most humanizes us, it is quite likely that they come from inadequate or poorly formed homes, where the parents were not interested or worried about stimulating and helping them in the acquisition of speech, this being, sometimes or most of the time, the cause of the speech defect or disorder, and these, by not expressing themselves normally, are the target of ironies, rejection, of "pity" or "compassion", going through tensions and frustrations that negatively affect the development of their personality and social adjustment.

Therefore, the adequate development of language in children enables the harmonious development of their personality, constituting a valuable instrument or means for learning and social integration. But, when there are defects, the child tends to present developmental maladjustments, generating certain behavioral-mental reactions such as shyness, feelings of inferiority, isolation and frustrations that, in short, lead to unhappiness.

What happens when there are defects in the tongue?
This question leads us to question ourselves in an extreme way, what would happen if we could not talk with our partner, children or other people? What would happen if they were accusing you of being a terrorist and you could not say that it was not true? And if you were sick, what if you couldn't say what hurts or how you feel?

All these questions make us aware of how important and essential the tongue is in the lives of human beings. It is with it that we can communicate, inform ourselves, read and understand, work and learn everything related to our life. However, when there are defects or disorders in this quality, there are serious interferences and limitations in the development and psychological adjustment of the affected person to their social environment.

This is the case, for example, of stutterers, for whom the defect not only constitutes an impediment to speech, but also to their lives, since it prevents them from following their educational and vocational aspirations and their development and social reciprocity.

To better understand and assess the consequences of a speech defect, let's look at the case of a 23-year-old young man who came to a psychological consultation due to his stuttering.

He states the following:

"(In a restaurant ...) ... I wanted a coffee and a tasty cake that was displayed on the counter, but I asked for a tea and a bread ... because I knew that if I tried to say those others Words would stutter a lot and I didn't want the lady who was attending me to feel sorry for me ... I hate bread alone ...

Since I was a child I isolated myself from my schoolmates for fear that they would make fun of me ... I have no friends who consider me ..., I have never had a girlfriend because of my defect."

In this story we can realize that the defect is not only a speech impediment, but is also a serious limitation for his development in life, since this prevents him from freely expressing what he wants, inducing frustration and social isolation.

This painful situation is rarely understood by normal people. Daily activities, such as answering the phone, asking or answering, talking to any other person, etc., constitute for subjects with this defect a source of deep concern, restlessness and tension, even becoming a true "nightmare". For them, everything goes well as long as they do not speak, but it is enough for them to know that they have to talk so that everything falls apart, tension and "panic" surface, blocking all aspects of their personality, hiding as a result of this in tics and tricks. I do not know if you know the story of the bullfighter named Belmonte, who was a stutterer, he preferred to face the worst of the bulls, the most ferocious miura.

According to these references, can we still doubt the importance of speaking well? Not really! Speaking well and with a good voice is the best quality that a person can have in a world like the one we live in. This allows him to communicate, feel active and useful to his peers; that is, to be much more human, since you can think, say what you feel and think, understand and help others using language.

The tongue and verbal language functions
Language fulfills a number of important functions in the life of human beings:

a) Communicative function: The primary function of language is communication. Human beings have a vital need to relate and this is possible thanks to language.

b) In this communication process, speech constitutes the decisive instrument of communication and social interrelation.

c) Cognitive function: Language also has a cognitive function; that is, it is a powerful instrument for learning and abstraction. Thanks to language we can project ourselves from the concrete to the abstract, from the proximal to the distal.

With the position of this quality, a human can elaborate his first elementary abstractions and concepts, with which he will understand and dominate his environment.

But, when there is a defect with the tongue, the person involved will have difficulties to abstract and, as such, it becomes a handicap for active performance and other cognitive activities.

a) Instrumental function to satisfy immediate needs: Verbal language allows to satisfy immediate needs such as hunger, thirst, shelter and is the most dietary and effective means to ask for help or assistance in situations of risk or danger. Without this quality we would perish.

b) Personal function: Man, through verbal language, can express his opinions, feelings, motivations, personal points of view and aspirations, sharing feelings, ideals and fantasies with others.

c) Informative function: The tongue allows us to obtain information about what is happening around us and in the world in which we live, contributing to the solution of problems, anticipating and adapting to changes. In this way, the tongue allows us to live more satisfactorily.

d) Adaptive function: The verbal language or speech allows the individual to adapt adequately and competently to the social environment. That is, it facilitates the adjustment and self-realization of the person, which translates psychologically into well-being or discomfort. The discomfort occurs precisely because of speech defects, constituting a limitation for life, as occurs with those affected by stuttering.

e) Regulatory function of behavior: Language has an important function as a regulator of the individual's behavior through internal language and, also, a "controlling" function on the behavior of others, through external language. This allows the child, like the adult, to establish and maintain social relationships.

These are, among others, the most important functions of tongue and verbal languages, characterized by being a valuable instrument of communication and thought.

Chapter Four

ANTAGONISTS OF THE HUMAN BODY

In medicine, when we refer to everything that is disease, war terms are depopulated: we talk about "fighting" the problem, "fighting" against the pathology, using the "therapeutic paraphernalia" in an exhausting "battle" for health. Here then is that Medicine becomes the strategy of "conquering" that primary and undisputed good which is health.

A misleading metaphor
In this war perspective, however, the body is no longer perceived as part of the patient, but becomes a battlefield, where doctor and disease collide, while the interested subject becomes a helpless spectator able only to witness what is a conflict decisive for his fate.

To understand how this perception came about, the reflection of Norman Doidge, psychiatrist winner of important literary prizes for his best seller "The infinite brain", illustrates how this vision is partly the result of the discoveries of the twentieth century, which led to the absolute centrality of the brain in the performance of many functions.

The discovery of his control of the body has led to the belief that everything happens in the brain, to the point of considering it almost as an entity in its own right with respect to the body. Consequently, the body would be nothing more than a mere appendage of the brain, a simple executor of it and the structure within which it is stored.

A one-to-one relationship
Such a conception of the human body is limiting and does not allow us to grasp the profound relationship that distinguishes the link between the brain and the rest of the organism: there is a continuous and one-to-one communication, guaranteed by the dense network of neurons present within the whole organism. This ensures that the exchange of information between inside and outside is constant and that body and mind are able to influence each other. The discoveries of recent years, precisely with regard to the neuronal networks distributed in the body, have led to the identification of networks that are so dense and organized that they can be defined as "brains."

In this regard, see:
The gut: our second brain sensitive to emotions the heart: our third brain with a powerful electromagnetic field. In this way the perception of the human body as a mere effector loses its thickness: the intertwining with the nervous system is so dense that it makes no sense to try to separate them.

A step back to move forward

Hippocrates believed that the body was the most important medicine. It was believed, in fact, that the body had its own therapeutic abilities and, as a patient and doctor, acting according to nature, was to elicit them, thus guaranteeing healing. The Hippocratic perception of medicine was holistic and was human-centered.

Paraphrasing Medicus, a film that conveys a different perception of the Doctor than today, the principle is that one should not take care of the disease, but of the person who has the disease. This is the key to hoping for the best results.

This is the message also conveyed by better known masterpieces such as Patch Adams:

"If you cure a disease you win or lose, if you treat a person, I guarantee you that in that case, you will win whatever outcome the therapy has" and *"The point is that to become doctors, we must treat the patient as well the illness. We have to dive into people, navigate the sea of humanity."*

So, if we take care of the person in his entirety, we understand how his organism - the body - is an integral part that cannot be ignored: it is a very sophisticated machine, which works incessantly to guarantee each of us the best possible level of well-being.

Precisely from the knowledge of its responses to different conditions (knowledge still far away in its totality) an optimal approach to the disease can be born: when we talk about the human body we are dealing with its laws which often do not correspond to that rationally one could think intuitively.

Moreover, the recent scientific discoveries are helping us to understand the incredible potential of the human body, first of all neuroplasticity, or the ability that the brain possesses to modify its own structure and functioning in response to mental activity and experience. And perhaps the most peculiar aspect of the efforts of neurology is how more and more doctors (and Dr. Norman Doidge returns to be illuminating in this regard), to make the most of the potential of neuroplasticity, are seeking a marriage between Western neuroscience and practices of oriental medicine - knowledge that has always placed at its center the joint action of energy and mind in healing.

At that point, one wonders if looking back is really a going back or if sometimes it is essential to turn around and become aware of past traditions in order to hope for better progress. One certainty remains: man, and the body he inhabits, remains the fulcrum of every medicine that aims at the well-being and health of man himself. The body, in this case, becomes an ally. Ally, because it is the first tool that each of us has at his disposal to get to know each other: educating oneself to listen to one's body can become a crucial aspect in the path of daily health.

What it really means to listen to your body? It is a path of knowledge, and like every path it presents a certain gradualness. It is important to get to know each other in everyday life, to learn to decipher the simplest sensations and then understand what is happening. Learning to know when you are full is the key, for example, to avoid overeating and avoid unnecessary stomach pain and - in the long run - weight gain.

Learning to feel when thirsty allows you to drink more frequently and stay hydrated. Knowing when your body is tired can become the tool for going to bed earlier in the evening rather than abusing coffee. What seem like trifles can become a valid help in everyday life and in solving those problems that are secondary to an inappropriate conduct that often imposes itself on us. Big results can be achieved in small steps. And that same knowledge of one's own body can be crucial in managing the disease, as no one can know the tricks to improve one's well-being as the person concerned. This is what it means to have your body as an ally: from respect for it comes the respect for one's person.

Germs/Diseases
Viruses, bacteria, pathogens, microbes… The tendency is quickly to amalgamate. Our hands carry 80% of infections. Our body does not have one, but three types of enemies. Diseases are caused either by viruses, bacteria or fungi. Enemies, who feed and reproduce differently.

Germs are present everywhere in our environment. Germs are the cause of most illnesses and infections. They are invisible to the naked eye. Viruses and bacteria attach themselves to surfaces and are dependent on exterior movement for their own movements. Fungi can be volatile and "catch" in the air. The lifespan of germs depends on their own nature, but also on the environment in which they are found.

A friction, a handshake, a touch, are enough to move germs from one place to another and from one body to another. Like all living things, germs need an environment conducive to their survival. As a priority, they therefore seek to attach themselves to surfaces on which they will find food and conditions that suit them (humidity, temperature, etc.).

Carrying a germ on you does not necessarily make you sick. We can very well have bacteria on our hands, without them generating an infection in our body. But, we can still transmit them to those around us by direct or indirect contact. An infection may start in a person even though it did not start in the person who passed the germ to them.

The three types of germs
Bacteria are microorganisms. That is to say that they are living beings which are made up of one or more cells. For example, some ear infections, tonsillitis and diarrhea are caused by bacteria.

Fungi are also microorganisms, made up of one to several cells. Their way of multiplying is particular. They release their spores into the environment (air, water, surfaces). These spores can reproduce autonomously (asexual reproduction), or they may need contact with a similar spore to become a new fungus (sexual reproduction). Itching of the scalp, feet or mucous membranes can be caused by fungi.

A third type of germ is the cause of many diseases. These are viruses. Nasopharyngitis, influenza and most tonsillitis are caused by viruses. These entities are not microorganisms, they are not made up of cells. Not having their own mechanism for producing energy like a bacterial cell does, they are dependent on the outside. Thus, viruses can only live and reproduce inside the cells of a living being (man, animals, plants or microorganisms). They are constantly trying to colonize cells to feed and multiply.

What happens when the body attacks itself?
Tiredness, difficulty sitting up, swollen limbs and bleeding, these are some of the many and varied symptoms that may be announcing the suffering of different autoimmune diseases, when the body's defenses become their attackers. Due to the low specificity of its symptoms, the diagnosis involves difficulties and can be delayed: a compelling reason to go to the doctor at the slightest suspicion. In these diseases, early diagnosis is crucial to avoid irreparable damage, even in young people.

Autoimmune diseases are those disorders that consist of making defenses (or immunity) against ourselves (hence the prefix "auto"), so that our immune system stops working as a pure defensive system - and harmless to the human body and becomes your enemy. This means that, instead of making defenses against pathogenic microorganisms that invade the body, they make antibodies that are directed against the cells of our own body and damage them.

The list of autoimmune diseases is extensive; more than 100 have already been identified. These include known diseases such as fibromyalgia, multiple sclerosis, celiac disease or Crohn's disease. But also others, which are perhaps less well known by the population, such as pernicious anemia, rheumatoid arthritis, Behçet's disease, antiphospholipid syndrome, Sjögren's syndrome, scleroderma, vitiligo, different types of vasculitis, inflammatory myopathies or myasthenia gravis. Some diseases affect a single organ, such as diabetes mellitustype 1 or juvenile diabetes, while others affect several of them (multi-organ or systemic), such as systemic lupus erythematosus (SLE).

Chapter Five

HUMANS

You have them too, like everyone else. It is a nuisance to make them protagonists, but in this entry it touches: Who are your adversaries and what to do with them?

Let's see if the little pleasant time that we are going to spend thinking about who opposes your interests is of any use and that you are happy. Because that's just the figure of the enemy. The upset begins.

Your 'antagonist' is someone who opposes your interests, either because it collides with theirs or because they have something personal against you. He hates you.

The enemy wants your bad, in contrast to the friend, who is who feels good when you are well.

We may not all have friends. But enemies, yes. Of those we always have.

Why say this?

Because, to be friends with someone, you need to build the relationship (from respect and trust), share interests or hobbies ... In short, work on it. Friendship is very beautiful, but it is a relationship that must be taken care of. If you don't take care of it, you can lose it.

It's easier with enemies. You don't have to do anything to have them.

Sometimes a person takes it with you and you are fatal to them without eating or drinking it. He finds out that you are from a football team other than his and he already has bad will on you.

Other times, in the fight for his own interest, he finds you in the middle ... And he takes you ahead or crushes you, as he sees fit. You have something you want. Or he sees you as a threat that separates him from his goal.

A real threat. Or a threat that is only in your head.
The possibilities are many. But no effort is required on your part either. One day you wake up and you see the destruction that he has done to you, the very nice one. And maybe then you find out that he was your enemy. But then, there are other chances that you don't have a bigger enemy than yourself?

- **Self**
In many of our experiences, we have felt abused and humiliated, and we think we got past that when it is not that simple.

Over time, this abuse disappears, but we start to exercise it against ourselves without really being aware of it.

This is where we need to realize how we really are. People with low self-esteem, full of insecurities, frustrations, fears, guilt ...

If you find it very difficult to value yourself, accept yourself, and recognize that you are capable of achieving everything that others have already achieved and achieved, you are surely becoming your own enemy.

You can choose to be your enemy or not
Your worst enemy is not other people, but what is on your mind. How is it possible? How can we become our own enemy?

All the criticisms that you can receive, the humiliations, the opinions, the judgments that you must make on yourself... All of this, you can accept them or not.

This decision-making power is within you. Do you think you deserve it, really? Do you agree with what others are saying?

Taking on something just to be accepted by others only fuels low self-esteem and that inner enemy.

It is obvious that being surrounded by diverse opinions makes you doubt who you really are. So, it is necessary to distance yourself from these people in order to be able to reflect on who you really are. Once you know it, you can face these opinions and judgments much more confidently.

How to stop being your own enemy?
- Accept yourself and be sure of who you really are.
- Question any negative messages that come to you.
- Learn to make mistakes.

Don't try to please everyone.
It's hard to stop being your own enemy, but it's within reach. You need to be confident in who you are and not let others dictate your conduct.

You have to start seeing mistakes not as burdens or shame, but as experiences that can be learned and then done better.

Everyone is wrong, but you feel humiliated. Know that there is no learning without errors. We learn more from mistakes than we think.

Who are you?
This is a very simple question, but it is difficult to answer. Do you know who you really are? If so, why do other people's criticism affect you so much?

You need to learn not to compare yourself to others, to be confident in yourself, and not to get carried away by what others may say. You are unique, extraordinary and irreplaceable, with flaws but also with qualities.

Trust, believe in yourself, and don't allow yourself to be how others want you to be. Being yourself will help you achieve the happiness we all dream of.

Your decisions are the ones that will mark your life from today. Who will decide in your life? You or the others?

Be a little selfish with yourself and stay away from what people say. Your life is yours, you alone decide how to live it.

Think that the confidence you have in yourself will allow you to move forward, to test, to experiment. If you don't trust yourself, insecurities will arise.

Ask yourself where you are heading your life. Want to be so perfect that you can't do it anymore? Perfection is by no means the right answer.

Be natural, try to improve yourself, make mistakes, learn and live the way you want. Free yourself from everything that is said to you, which blocks you and paralyzes you. Be free from all of this and move on. Never allow yourself to be your own enemy.

Okay. Now you know this and you're obviously prepared not to be your own enemy. Still, there might be a problem. Someone, or people might just hate you more.

- **Others**
  "The man is a wolf for the other man", affirmed the philosopher Thomas Hobbes to remember the tendency of the human beings to fight the one against the other.

Of course, the wolfish gaze of the gentleman sitting across from me in the airport boarding area bites. "Get away, flock of sheep," he seems to say in his wordless language. Perhaps he is having a bad day or he is one of those aggressive toxic guys who circulate with his loaded hostility submachine gun, which is certain, is that the man in question has decided that his frustration at the flight delay is his neighbor's fault. He dislikes everyone!

Has it happened to you that, sometimes, you get up on the wrong footing and everything bothers you? Have you ever perceived that others are superficial and stupid? Have you felt like a weirdo for hating humanity? Do you want "to stop the world that to allow you to get off"? If you have answered yes to any of these questions, do not worry, the most likely explanation is that you are a victim of stress, fatigue or the feeling of not being understood.

"To fall badly or well" is an attitude that serves to regulate the proximity that we are willing to allow to other human beings. It is something intuitive, a sensation based on details as minute as the clothes they wear, how they speak or sustained by prejudices as serious as their gender, their skin color or their creed. The brain warns from the depths of the limbic system: the amygdala is activated because someone gives it a bad feeling.

Negativist Bias
This hatred of humanity is consolidated thanks to the power of the tongue. There are ways of getting hooked on negative thoughts that make us approach others in an unconstructive way.

By virtue of the so-called negativity bias, negative expressions grab the mind's attention and produce an immediate emotional response while positive ones don't have it so easily. A simple "okay" doesn't generate much enthusiasm, while "it's wrong" hits us right away.

Christine Liebrecht, from the University of Tilburg, and her team published their research on this linguistic gap in the

'Giornal of Language and Social Psychology'. In the study, the subjects exchanged opinions about a restaurant. Those who thought the food was good weighed less than those who criticized it because it was bad. Surely the finding does not surprise you, just read the comments of others on any social network, in general, negative words make a greater impression than positive ones.

These hostile comments towards humanity serve to quickly charge us with reasons and justify the rejection of people that we do not want to overlook under any circumstances.

When we consider that the problems come from others, we end up disliked by everything they do. For highly dependent personalities, temporary negativity towards others is the only way to allow themselves time and space: while the anger lasts, they can stay away.

Mirror Effect
The problem arises when judging our peers as unworthy people lasts too long and becomes a habit. In these situations, the fact that you dislike others can hide the fear of being rejected and, as a compensation mechanism, you previously reject yourself.

Sigmund Freud referred to this behavior as "the expression of the defense mechanism of projection": you avoid feeling emotional discomfort in yourself and you put yourself on another person (you project yourself).

Our own emotion comes to be seen as something belonging to the other. In short, hating someone means hating in their image something that we have ourselves (positive emotions are also projected as in falling in love).

Jacques Lacan was a French psychoanalyst who spoke of the mirror stage, a stage that occurs in children between six and eighteen months. These infants, seeing themselves in the mirror for the first time complete, feel joy. This is the moment of the formation of the ego of the subject.

What Lacan highlights is that the recognition of one's own mirror image occurs with the help of and in relation to another similar one. From that moment on we get to know each other through relationships with others that thus become our mirrors (and we mirrors of our fellow men). Therefore, when we meet someone we really do not like, we must ask ourselves what this person has to do with me, what bothers me so much and why, before assuming that the world is against us.

Envy and Resentment
Sometimes it is the rancor and resentment that do not heal and persist in the present that make others lazy, superficial, insensitive, ignorant or careless and by judging them in such a way we have a free hand to unload on them our bad vibes.

Others, we cannot allow ourselves to do the same as that person or, we simply want what the other has and that unleashes anger and frustration. Instead of acknowledging the unhealthy envy and transforming it into an appreciation or a proactive emotion, we tend to generate a negative feeling towards which we believe makes us feel bad.

When you dislike everyone, think about these aspects because perhaps you are putting your own ghosts and fears in others in facing life, or perhaps, you hope that someone will rescue you and take care of you as when you were a child.

Human beings need others and it is true that sometimes beyond our state we can run into difficult, selfish or narcissistic personalities, but the important thing in these cases is that we can manage our emotions without clouding our judgment.

Chapter Six

DEATH: THE DESTINATION OF THE HUMAN BODY

Death is too exact; all the reasons are on its side. Mysterious for our instincts, it is drawn, before our reflection, limpid, without prestige and without the false attractions of the unknown." - EM Cioran, Breviary of Rot.

Every passing day, man is growing to become more complicated than this world, his world and he are in a constant differentiation and tangle. Its biological constitution and the variability of its environment have led to development and physiological and neurological transformations with immeasurable levels of complexity. Such complexity weaves a network over all spheres and areas of man from which nothing escapes.

Under this pathos, death has become more complicated, it is no longer a simple event, as our Neanderthal ancestors thought (Morin 2000: 113-115), now it is something that is embedded in the very consciousness and bio-ontological constitution of man. There is a recognition of mortality and transcendence, in whatever form. That is, the life of man, from the moment in which he became conscious - true original sin, has revolved around death, even to the point of affirming, as Heidegger tells us, that being-is-for-the-death (Heidegger 1987: 276).

In this sense, we can say together with Camus, that all the fundamental and serious problems of Philosophy and Anthropology they refer to death. Every philosophical (and anthropological) attempt to find meaning in life and man falls back on a reflection on death (Camus 1996: 9).

The following work tries to give some insights on the different transfigurations of death that have occurred to this day. Death continues to be a constitutive phenomenon of our reality, although it is banalized and seen as the simple end of a life, like a breakdown or a disease, just as our consumer societies do. However, the consequences of "living," death and interpreting it under the logic of consumerism and hegemonic commercialism are self-destructive, pernicious and in many cases, irreversible.

Death has been reduced to a scientific fact, a simple positive fact subject to observation and experimentation. These representations of death are intrinsic to the subjective movements of societies, our post-industrial era radiates and confers particular signs and meanings to death. Death becomes the representation of the machine that does not work, that is damaged, becomes the limit and fails of the production and re-production of the human being, of social systems and of the great economic machinery.

The last anthropological limit of human existence
"If I kill myself it will not be to destroy myself but to rebuild myself." - A. Artaud, Van Gogh: the suicide by society.

Throughout history, death has been present in one way or another in man's thought, either as an event of social, religious, political, etc. (Evans-Pritchard 1973), as a record in memory as an abstraction or as a philosophical or scientific reflection.

In Anthropology, these different ways of thinking about death converge, together with the different sciences of man. In this sense, death, being a multidimensional phenomenon inherent to man, is studied from an anthropological perspective. That is, every phenomenon is studied from its fundamental unit, and man is this fundamental unit. In order to understand what we are, we have to study death, and in order to understand death, we have to study man. Death, then, appears to us as a "subject-object" of study, pathos by which humanity has traced its existence.

Anthropology claims to be the most ambitious science par excellence, it wants to embrace man from all his angles, seeing him from an infinity of raw materials; but like any ambitious project, it fell short. Knowledge, science, anthropology, cannot go beyond our life, our senses, our language, our world, and only through this combination of elements can we form any system of thought or representation. Death is presented as that limit from which we cannot escape. We cannot know, know, much less explain, what is there after death. Ancestral, biblical question, prehistoric, that continues and will continue to reverberate in our heads, fluttering chaotically like a butterfly in the back of our minds. Perhaps it will be selfish death that does not want to reveal the secrets of life to us, or complex life that does not want us to know the secrets of death. However, death inscribed in life, but also overflowing it, expanding as rapidly as time. Death encoded in man (Morin 1999), part of the primordial component that sustains, bases and forms life. Endless fundamental cycle from which all cycles start.

Death is the great project; it is the totalizing end. In death the consciousness of man ends, dissolving into the unknown. Death is, in part, metaphysical, but it is also an event, randomness, focus, accident, death is Hegelian, but it is also Nietzschean; it is dialectical and eternal return at the same time. It is the zero point of our world, it is the moment that we cannot grasp, of which Ernst Bloch speaks. Death is the infinite horizon that escapes us at every moment, synthesized disorder and order, a dislocated fragment that is diluted in history, in life, in our being.

Death is presented to us as biological, but also as cultural, it is empirical data, but also symbolic, it is the most human trait (Morin 1999: 13), MORIN would say. We are the only living beings on earth who reflect on death, and not just death, but usefulness of life, itself.

Although this is more important - our own death is the next step that leads us to a new maturity, knowing that we are dying and that others are also going to die. No animal has the ability to make its own death conscious, it only dies, there is no death for animals, but that instinct, which, like us, is biogenetically established: the survival instinct. The animal is not aware that it is dying moment by moment, that each day that passes inevitably approaches, that at any moment it can unexpectedly break into our life, ironic? or can life also break into death?

Life bursts into death at all times, in the constant eternal return of the instant and the unrepeatable creative act; thus, some die so that others can live. In ancient times, the dead were those who had life, preceptors, advisers and guides of the living. Dead or alive, man serves and will serve life.

"Man not only mythically appropriates the law of death-resurrection to found his own immortality, but also strives to magically use the life-engendering force that constitutes death, for his own vital purposes." (Morin 1999: 121)

The death that gives us life, makes us aware of our finitude, of our ephemeral and transitory state, maintains and delimits existence, death distinguishes us, without it we are nothing or nobody. The main characteristic is that of being human: our dignity. In this sense, all subjectivity is traversed by death, as well as all objective limitations of human practice.

Since man became aware of this phenomenon, the great myths appeared, the majestic legends that gave life to hominid history. Death is, duplication, the image of the other. The dead, in prehistoric societies, possess food, weapons, clothes, desires, thoughts, motivations; the dead are doubles of the living and vice versa. Death is rebirth, an endless cycle, as in the Christian and Buddhist religions, although each of them interprets death-rebirth differently, even in a contradictory way.

It is evident that we do not know about death, we only know about our attitude towards it. We only know about pains, agonies, processes, phases, stages, not of death itself, but of dying; absolute death, sudden death, apparent death, what difference does it make, we don't know anything. So, agony is the medical, psychological, sociological condition of people who are in the final phase of a disease or severe trauma, it is the last moment of existence. We know what happens just before it bursts into consciousness and vanishes everything. We only know the biological data immanent to the material body.

In this way, we must see death in its complete nakedness, decontaminated from us, unmasked; we have to take away that "personality", or rather, stop conceiving it as a person (mask). A mask built by society and the superego. We must stop seeing it outside of us, and see it inside, not as that ghost, double, spirit or soul that reflects our own being, but as a reality, as a constituent element of us and our world.

This mask arises from the impossibility of making the experience of one's own death conscious, therefore, consciousness will have to adopt a representation of death given by the society in which the subject is inserted. In this sense, we only know our death thanks to the death of others since death annihilates the means and the senses that human beings have to verify their existence. For consciousness, death is the last anthropological limit of existence.

The great German poet Rainer Maria Rilke underlines the advantages of appropriating death, becoming familiar with it, which does not mean becoming obsessed with it. In reality, anonymous death, which the consumer society cultivates, only leads to anonymous, depersonalized, dehumanized life. It is a great alienation to never think about death, live as if it does not exist, or only think about it in terms of life insurance, which is actually death insurance. Some seek in vain to hide their fear in fun, flight and escapism.

According to Rilke, if we are afraid of death it is because we have not known how to cultivate the death that each one of us carries within. Humanizing death is understanding and living its meaning. The question about the meaning of death arises urgently and inescapably. By presenting death as the last and the end of life, it gives it its ultimate meaning and purpose.

Every human being has to take on a great task, take charge of his life, and learn to live. Death prompts us to live a more authentic existence: accept our finitude, appreciate our itinerant condition, relativize the accumulation of goods and social functions, disqualify selfishness and the desire for profit, not to waste time, but to enjoy the seriousness of life - present moment and task. We seek to explore the face of death and discover what it teaches us with its silence and silence. The celebration of the Day of the Dead helps us to remember, to bring to our hearts, the memory of our loved ones.

Many ancient and modern thinkers point out that philosophy, the love of wisdom, has among its main functions learning or teaching how to die. Deep down, learning to die is learning to live, which implies giving life a purpose, a direction and a meaning, which goes beyond the instinct for self-preservation and cultivates the instinct for self-improvement.

Man does not limit his performance to satisfying basic survival needs, but rather seeks to confer value and meaning on his life and death. Even in moments when life seems to lose its meaning, in times of crisis and decadence, anxiety, restlessness and anguish appear as paradoxical witnesses that the search for meaning, value and the demand for an end and an order, they never disappear from the human mind and heart.

In fact, death is an event that raises legitimate questions about the being and the work of man. Death is not just a big question mark that encompasses all of life, but a reality that raises many unknowns.

Apparently, it is convenient to consider the framework of the human condition, its itinerant vocation, since death is on the way. But what is death? Is it something specific, or rather an ingredient of life? His face is enigmatic, but also multifaceted: death is something distant and close, friend and foe, natural and unnatural, and it performs a critical function for man and for society.

We must bear in mind our mortal condition, as travelers, as passing through this world, pilgrim beings who always glimpse death on the horizon, which helps us to walk wisely on earth.

The Spanish poet Jorge Manrique uses the metaphor of the river: "our lives are the rivers / that go to the sea / that is dying". The rivers are for Pascal, roads that walk. The essence of the river is not to stagnate, always flow, always run, precipitously in the rapids, calmly in the backwaters, but always, continuously, constantly, advance.

Is it possible to have a rest, as the Roman epitaph suggests: Stop, walker! Stop in space, not in time, the itinerant condition always leads us to move forward. In any case, the human being does not have permanent residence here, nor is he on this earth as at home, "to be is to be on the road": not to be dormant, always to move forward, to be attentive and vigilant to the signs of the road and the risks that it implies.

For the pilgrim, it would be absurd if the path led to nothingness, if it led to annihilation. The goal, the end, the culmination of the path would not be the what is expected, it would be meaningless. It is important to be in search of an end, beyond which it is not worth prolonging the journey. Be open to novelty and the sense of the invisible. The goal, however, illuminates the entire path: hope shines in the chiaroscuro of faith.

Chapter Seven
_____

THE WAY AND THE HUMAN BODY

The Way gives birth to one
One gives birth to two
Two gives birth to three
Three gives birth to the universe
Everything that carries negative holds positive
Combined, they are in harmony
The human hates orphans, widow, and useless ones
But the king sees himself as that
Therefore, his thoughts increase but also decrease
And then his thoughts decrease but also increase
The words that others and I promote are
"Violent man has brutal death!"
That is the main point I recommend.
Chapter 42 - The Book of Ethics

We see the numbers one, two, and three recurring in the poem above, which are easily relatable to everyone. However, in this poem, one, two, and three are not in a numerical context. According to the Way - one implies the universe, two- Yin and Yang, and three- the Heavens. Earth and its Inhabitants (people) who multiply all things, comprising of Yin and Yang, which produces Harmony. Our world is full of harmony, the fruits of Yin and Yang.

Since one is recognized as the universe, it is sensible to make this correlation. First, with a question, what does this Taoism have to do with the body? The Way - Tao is not practiced without an aim, and the reason why the Way is existent will no longer be possible if the body is absent.

Without the body, harmony, balance, yin, and yang, and other fundamentals, which are discussed in the subsequent chapters will not be achievable. The Way seeks to reconstruct the body to the earliest energy (Qi) felt and enjoyed at creation (free flow), so that the body is no longer a means to an end but the end itself. The body becomes the Universe (One).

Stanza four of the poem in Chapter 42 - The Book of Ethics says, "Three gives birth to the Universe." Do you see the connection? Three is the earth and its inhabitants (You). It means You give birth to the universe. This makes sense because only the You-niverse can birth the universe. It is a fact that the Way centers on the body; therefore, it should be treated with utmost priority to harmonize the world. The body is a transporter of feelings, thoughts, actions, representation, and expression of a practice, religion, ideology, school of thought.

According to Tao, the body is underrated when perceived as a physical container that houses other components or a spirit-material (flesh) component. It is revered as a means of journeying into Immortality, which you must understand maximum function. The body's symbolism is not just bringing various practices, meanings, and observations together but, most importantly, it gives full expressions to these perspectives. Through the diverse connotations, the body is put up to its full potential and is maximized by the practice, harnessing, and cultivation of The Way.

Nature is quiet
Strong wind does not blow the whole morning
Heavy rain does not fall all-day
Why? Heaven and earth!
If heaven and earth can't do it
How can humans do it?
One with the Way
Then becomes one with the Way
One with Virtue
Then becomes one with Virtue
One who loses the Way and the Virtue
Then becomes one with loss
When one is one with the Way
The Way welcomes one
When one is together with the Virtue
The Virtue is always there
When one is together with loss
The loss also follows one
One who is disbelieved
It should not be believed.
Chapter 23 - The Book of Ethics

Nature is a fundamental of Tao, and it preaches returning to the source, which means different things, particularly returning to the original body - emotional energy and good health. We lose our golden/original body as we grow and evolve due to stress, trauma, depression, bad eating habits, and the likes. The Way is after a system to reverse the deterioration of the body to flow with nature and function from its original state freely.

The origin of the human body; Science or religion?

The religious perspective about man's origin is the belief that divine creation is responsible for life and the universe, contrary to scientific consensus that supports a natural means of evolution.

Since evolutionary phenomena have been described in astronomy, geology, and biology, creationists (those who believe in the religious part of human origin) have maintained controversy in this regard, because the scientific explanation of these phenomena is not compatible with their interpretation of religious texts. The debate raises important political issues, in particular in matters of education, scientific research, freedom of opinion, and beliefs.

Creationist currents show great diversity, from those who support fixism by developing a theory of theistic nature ("Jeune-Terre creationism" and "Vieille-Terre") to those with more deistic positions who embrace the transformist theory (hypothesis of the intelligent design and directed panspermia).

The Creationism Young-Earth reads the Bible or the Koran as scientific and historical books, conveying the belief that the story of the creation of the universe, as provided by religious texts, gives a literally accurate description of the origin of the Universe. This literal interpretation of texts like Genesis is based on the conviction that these texts were "dictated by God" as absolute, definitive, and indisputable truths (the case of certain Protestant churches, the majority in the Bible Belt of the United States). This current of thought is generally associated with the rejection of any idea of biological and geological evolution.

Most monotheistic religious traditions (Judaism, Christianity, and Islam) postulate the creation of the world by a supreme God. The fundamentalist reading is refused by the majority of current Christian Churches, which favor a hermeneutical reading.

For Catholics, the creation of the universe by God is not in itself opposed to evolution: creation is above all the relationship between creatures and a Creator, their first principle.

Creationism is not, however, restricted to currents that interpret religious texts literally, but also includes Old-Earth creationism which admits that the universe is well over 6000 years; the partisans of intelligent design, of currents which admit aspects of the theory of evolution but exclude a man from it; theistic evolution which admits that the evolution of species takes place but that it is directed or influenced by divinities or a Creator who would give birth to the universe, to the living and to the mechanisms allowing them then to evolve by them.

According to creationism, everything starts from God. The stance of creationism suggests certain philosophical dilemmas:

How did the world come to be? How is it possible for something to be created out of nothing?

There is a metaphysical principle that states, "nothing comes out of nowhere." Therefore, if the universe, which encompasses everything that exists, had an origin, it would have arisen out of nowhere, nullifying the aforementioned principle. To overcome this contradiction, we would need to accept that the universe always existed. For creationism, this means that existence is given by God, who is eternal and has always existed.

As earlier said, creationism is often claimed to be opposed to Charles Darwin's theory of evolution. This scientist explained that all species, including humans, are derived from other species. This would therefore assume that man wasn't created out of nothing. On the other hand, creationists believe that each species is the fruit of an act of divine creation.

Taoist (Dao) perspective of the body

The human body is defined based on three terms:

One, ti/body meaning the physique; Two, xing/form means to form or being; Three, Shen/person implying the whole human; material and non-material. The body is a complicated term in Taoism due to its various contexts:

- The body and state: they are two microcosms related to each other and the macrocosm. The concept of microcosm-macrocosm states that humans are microcosms (smaller universe) which corresponds significantly to the macrocosm (large universe).

The big country seems to be located in low land
That is the gathering place of all species
The mother of all things
Females prevail over males due to their stillness
Take stillness as a low place
Therefore, if a big country is humble with a small country
Then it will conquer the small country
If a small country is modest with a big country
Then it will be protected by the big country
So staying below to get it
Or staying below to be protected
A big country wants to accommodate many people
The small country needs many people to accommodate
Each side gets what they want
So, the big country should learn to be humble.
Chapter 61 - The Book of Ethics

- The body and cosmos: this is based on the supernatural form of Laozi known as Laojun, the supreme Lord of Tao, including its Virtue. In the Scriptures, Transformation of Laozi and Opening of Heaven, the man, Laozi, is seen at the creation of the cosmos and reappearing throughout life in various bodily forms. Cosmos is taken to be his body.

- The body as a home for gods, celestial bodies, and spirits: in the book Laozi zhongjing, the description of deities who live in different body parts was explained as one supreme being in forms (Taoiyi). These deities perform a balance function in the viscera: liver, kidneys, lungs, spleen, and heart. In addition, they are the abode of unseen forces. The Heshang gong describes the hun soul as Yang, po soul as yin, essence as jing, spirit as Shen, with you residing in the five viscera.

Five colors make people's eyes blind
Five sounds make people's ears buzz
Five flavors make people's tongue lose taste
Chasing hunting horses makes people go crazy
Rare and precious possessions make one degrade
Sage prays for a full stomach
And yet there's nothing spectacular
Therefore, leave this and get that.
Chapter 12 - The Book of Ethics

- The body as a mountain and landscape: The five's: planets, sacred mountains, and viscera are related to wudi zhenfu (five emperors) in the Wushang biyao (Supreme Secret Essentials Book).

By keeping body and soul together
Is it possible to keep them apart?
Pay attention to breathe
To be soft
Can one become an infant?
With spiritual cleansing
Can the stain be gone?
Love people and rule country
The heaven gate opens and closes
Through everything
Can't we do anything?
We are born and raised
Instructions without possessions

Made without merit
Instruction without ruling
Such is the root of the Way.
Chapter 10 - The Book of Ethics

- The body related to Internal Alchemy: the major constituents of the internal state (breath, essence, spirit, shen). The focus is not the bodily form rather the loci (pivotal points) where energy is channeled from five points to achieve balance.

The Taoist View on Gender

Male-Female balance, otherwise known as yin and Yang, was formed in the 6th century by Lao Tzu, the Taoist scholar in Tao De Jing. His classical work was the stepping stone for respecting women. Several philosophies and ideologies allow the female to be discriminated against, ignored, or subjected.

Until just a few decades ago, scholars viewed women as simply passive participants in evolutionary change and limited themselves to relegating them to the role of giving birth, feeding, and caring for their young. While, on the contrary, men were described as responsible for many of the innovations that define us as humans, for example, the emergence of bipedal gait, brain enlargement, tool-making, cooperative communication, or symbolic representation.

Thus, it should not be surprising that research related to our evolution has, and still does, carry away the conventional sexist bias that has permeated the academic world and the models it produces for centuries.

However, in Taoism, women are dignified and given a chance to express themselves by being independent. In the history of

Tao, Wu Chengzhen is the first female master who applauded Yi Ching, the Chinese Classic on Gender equality. The awesomeness of balance, equality of yin and Yang (water and fire, good and bad, male and female, etc.) is elaborated, which were then in Chinese history, the best thing to happen in her words. According to Tao De Jing, the female body is related to the potency of Tao, illustrated as a divine gate bearing lives, a valley, and a power source.

Know the male and keep the female,
Making streams for people.
Making streams for people,
Virtue does not leave
Return to the childhood
Know the light and keep the dark,
Be an example for the world.
Be an example for the world,
Virtue does not leave
Return to infinite
Know the honour and keep the humiliation,
Make a cave for the world.
Make a cave for the world,
Virtue is full
Return to the rustic
Rustic is not divided
Sage uses it to provoke hundreds of officials
So, the great spell is not undercut.
Chapter 28 - The Book of Ethics

The yin (female) is concluded to be equivalent to the yang in both strength and Importance. We have to accept yin to understand Yang. They also ate interdependently and related to reproduction, and only in this is the oneness of the element achieved. Every individual has a touch of masculinity and femininity. The Way encourages the understanding and cultivation of yin to the extent of Yang.

The union of the human body and mind

This has always been a problem that keeps human beings arguing all the time. That is: Does the body control the mind or does the mind control the body? The philosophers participating in the debate have their own opinions, which can be roughly divided into two viewpoints: materialism and idealism.

The mind and body are not two incompatible aspects. Both the mind and the body are part of our life, and both are expressions of life. We should understand their relationship on the basis of seeing life as a whole.

Foreseeing one's own actions in advance is the most critical role of the soul. Knowing this, we can realize: how the mind controls the body - the mind sets the direction of the next action for the body.

If we don't have a direction to work hard, but only receive some scattered movement signals, it is useless. Since the mind can determine the direction of our actions, it occupies a pivotal position in life. At the same time, the mind is also affected by the body, the body is the executor of the action, and the mind can only exercise commanding powers within the scope of the body's abilities. For example, if the mind wants the body to run to the moon in the sky, it is nonsense unless it can overcome the limitations of the human body.

The horse and the horse rider is a good example. The horse rider can direct the horse to go, but he cannot specify the details precisely. It cannot be forced. It can only be guided. In the end, it will be decided by the horse.

Mankind's ability to foresee the future will definitely develop in the long term, and mankind will work hard for the goals set by itself in order to consolidate the important position of mankind in the environment.

By studying the meaning contained in the various expressions of the individual, find a suitable way to understand the object, and compare his goals with the goals of other people.

In most cases, the mind affects the body. When a person thinks about something in his head, he will work hard on the matter, and finally, give feedback to the body.

Everything has origin
At the beginning of everything is the mother of all
By keeping the mother, one knows the child
By knowing the child, one keeps the mother
Therefore, one should not be in danger for a lifetime
Close-lipped, breath held
Life is full
Open-lipped, always busy
Life is futile
Seeing hidden is bright

INSIGHTS TO BETTER LIVING

Hold strength is strong
Use Virtue to return to the Way
Do not let the body be in trouble
Thus, the Way is eternal.
Chapter 52 - The Book of Ethics

89

Chapter Eight

THE TAOIST VIEW ON DEATH

People are not afraid of death
Why use death to scare?
If it makes people always afraid
And if every criminal is caught and killed
So, who is left?
Killing is carried out by the executioner
Replace that person
Like replacing a woodcutter
Which rarely cuts hands?
Chapter 74 - The Book of Ethics

The Way explains how things are done naturally; the way plants grow, the way we breathe, the way water flows, etc. Transformation happens consistently in both humans and nature; hence, when individuals have insight into the natural way things occur, they will find it simple to accept pain, sorrow, grief, or joy and be unaffected by it. With understanding, the surge of emotions can be subdued. For instance, a family is preparing for an evening outing when a heavy downpour of rain begins. The children will naturally be unhappy and probably cry because they would be unable to go out while the parents having understanding do not get mad but see it as a natural cause. Zhuangzi, the ancient philosopher, stopped mourning when his wife died because he realized that it was a part of the change. Just as seasons come and go, death is such; the springtime, summer, the autumn, and winter. Hence, to mourn is going against the law of nature and acting oblivious. In the cycle of change and the Earth, life and death are embedded therein. We live to die and die to live. This is nature's way; plants grow, animals consume them (herbivores), other animals consume them (carnivores), man kills them, and we also die and are taken into the Earth where microbes feast on, making the soil fertile. The inability of a man to unbound himself from his classification of life and existence is why Grief is experienced; the dead and the living are alike. Death is inevitable, Man must die, yet his essence is permanent.

The theory of Zhuangzi is in line with Tao Te Ching (Daode-Jing). Man is to exist as a member of Nature worth other parts of and within Nature. It is only in freedom that he understands the Tao. Freedom from:

- Man's ideologies and intellectual bias.
- Emotional surge (insight into the way life is).
- Barriers are due to natural occurrences.

When we see death as transformation, not disappearance, we appreciate life better and see death as a drive.

The Concept of Death
We all remain a part of the Tao. We live as a constituent of Tao and die as a constituent of Tao.

- Based on yin-Yang theory, the transformation from being (existing) to not being (not existing) is death; change from Yang to yin. Nature sees no variation in life and death. Instead, a harmonization for balance is to be obtained. Death should be viewed as the same.

- We are taught to accept all things as essentials, whether good or bad. Death is part of the forces of eternity. Life and Death complement the Way.

The Concept of Afterlife

Newborn humans are pliable
When they are dead, they are stiff
Newly born trees are soft
When they are finished, they are complex and dry
So stiff and rigid represent death
Pliable and softness mean life
Strong and violent is the dead
Hard trees are cut
So hard and strong should be put under
Pliable and softness should be put above.
Chapter 76 - The Book of Ethics

- Life after death is indifferent; the same as it was while you were on Earth. They are One.

- Whatever you believed in before death is what is Incorporated. Do you believe in God or gods? You will be a part of them in your Afterlife.

Usually, the memories of our dead linger, and some persons may add that to their rituals to invoke and pay homage to their ancestry and memories, for example, the Qingming festival.

Chapter Nine

A LIFESTYLE FOR
A LONGER LIFE

The role of the body in spiritual enlightenment, longevity, balance, and harmony is indispensable. There is no way out without the body. The earlier you understand this and take the necessary action in preserving and maintaining your physique according to Nature's Way, the better you'd achieve.

A skilled plant is difficult to eradicate
A skilled grasp is difficult to slip
Virtue will be honored from generation to generation
By fixing Virtue in oneself, Virtue will be real
By fixing Virtue in the house, Virtue will have redundancy
By fixing Virtue in the village, Virtue will grow
By fixing Virtue in the country, Virtue will be in abundance
By fixing Virtue in the world, Virtue will be everywhere
So, by oneself that considers others
By one's house that considers other houses
By one's village that considers other villages
By one's nation that considers other nations
By one's people that consider other people
How do we know what people are? Thanks for that!
Chapter 54 - The Book of Ethics

Taoism does not see the body differently from the spirit because it believes that our actions create a spiritual impact.

- Purity -The body is kept in purity for the purpose of maintaining spiritual well-being. Purity is attained by avoiding specific kinds of nutritional choices and physical activity. Attributes that should be avoided are dishonesty, immorality, pride, etc.
- Meditation - It is a mandatory practice, and essential for achieving stillness, mindfulness, and boosting mental health.
- Breathing - Engaging in the various breath practices like qigong helps Taoist receive ch'i (energy).
- The flow of Energy - Ch'i can be generated, achieved, and fully harnessed by the right exercises, nutrition, and meditative practice.
- Martial arts - Original Taoist exercises like Tai Chi are encouraged.
- Diet -Not all crops and meat sources are permitted for consumption.

Improving body posture and food digestion

Taoist standing routine
Centuries ago, inside the Mount of China, the Taoist Monks attained a healthy life through posture and spine maintenance, a healthy and balanced diet, physical fitness routine coupled with martial arts prowess. Their show of balance and energy together with these features is known as Tensegrity.

Tensegrity
The term was formulated by Buckminster Fuller while working on his Geodesic Dome in the 1940's. This dome functions by joining and maintaining the balance between its components

tension and compression in contrast to a work that will stack its components upon themselves leading to the whole weight carried by the bottom.

This is applicable to the way we make our bodies function. It is in both manners either dumping the majority of one's weight on some joints or allowing an even distribution of the weight across all parts. The choice is yours.

Your body is a Tensegrity medium that maintains the spine for the functioning of other body systems.

Tensegrity and Birth
When a child is born, the muscles are still being developed. Think back to when you put your finger in a baby's hand and the reaction; tightening his hand around your finger with a subtle force caused by muscle and soft tissue movements (tensile), transmitted into the phalanges (compression) resulting in the tightening of the baby's hand.

Naturally, the muscular and skeletal systems work more effectively as the child grows older. Tensility moves up, down, sideways, to all parts and the body becomes stronger to walk, run, carry things and graduate to even more demanding activities. This push and pull is an avenue for the body to be massaged. Through this movement, the visceral organs like the liver, gastrointestinal organs, etc. are being exercised. When we make tensegrity the basis of our movement, our body systems particularly digestive and excretion will function maximally.

Why do we not experience tensegrity?
Sadly, many of us do not maintain this tensegrity and in a matter of time, our bodies move to stack. Hence, the lower

limbs and back take responsibility for carrying a major part of the body's weight and keeping the torso against tipping the pelvis (hips). Initially, the lower back and pelvic region are strong. However, due to (lack of use-synonym) the lower part of the abdomen gets weak.

After a period, the region from the navel, through the body's midsection, to the spinal cord, and the hip floor gets exhausted and (tight-synonym) leading to the Colon's inability to move and affecting excretion. The weakness of the colon is caused by friction in the lower limbs, abdomen, and pelvis. When challenges with excretion surface, it is no doubt that absorption will be affected.

What is the way out?
Our solution lies in returning to baby-like functioning. Make use of Nature's Way and blessing to our body; Tensegrity. The energy from the lower limbs (legs) to the abdomen has to be harnessed and grown. Block training is an easy method of understanding and grooming tensegrity founded by John Bracy (Master).

To strengthen your muscles, bring your body into alignment, and boost your digestive system, follow this Taoist standing routine for 300 seconds only!

1. Purchase a cinder block or a 6 inches thick wood (wood higher than the ground for you to stand with both feet shoulder apart).

2. Get on the block. Ensure your feet are straight (check if your second toe is straight) and relax your shoulders.

3. Quickly check the alignment of your body by ensuring your ears over shoulders, shoulders above hip, and hip above the ankle. Your knees should be slightly bent. Prevent your heels from bearing the weight.

4. Your jaw should be relaxed by allowing your teeth to touch, and not clenching them. The tip of your tongue should rest on your oral roof.

5. Locate a point to light a candle on the wall or space 6 feet from you and focus on it.

Standing for a period of 5-10 minutes daily is advisable for a start till you can increase. It may seem like you're doing nothing. In fact, you are working hard because inactive muscles are being used.

Shaky legs are common during the exercise and after it. Muscle soreness is also normal. Your denatured core muscles are being trained. Surfers seem to avoid denaturing because their muscles are pushed to ride the waves.

Block training is an activity that helps an individual attain balance and prevents the possibility of stressing the body leading to losing tensegrity. The legs are being strengthened together with the abdominal muscles and pelvis. In addition to enhancing balance and eliminating body tension, it boosts unison in the body systems.

In caring for others and worshiping god
There is nothing like restraint
Restraint begins with giving up one's will

*This belongs to Virtue gained from experience
If you store a lot of Virtue, nothing can be undone
If there is nothing one can't undo, then there's no restraint
If there is no restraint, then one can cure the country
Knowing the root of country treatment is long-lasting
That is called deeply-rooted, durable descent
That is the Way to live long and see throughout.
Chapter 59 - The Book of Ethics*

The purpose of Taoism is to boost the well-being and longevity of individuals. Diet has a major role in this mission. The ancestors of Taoism have endorsed and thoroughly scrutinized the Taoist diet. Though diet differs across generations, a meal of grains, vegetables, meat, and fruits is constant while water and tea are beverages. The pillar of Chinese culture is Taoism. According to the Chinese word for food, Yin Shi (beverages/food), they complement one another. The major prominent lineages are:

The Zheng Yi Dao lineage: allowed to eat anything except a few.

The Quan Zhen Dao: strict nutritional rules (no meat and alcohol).

Meals

1. Selecting ingredients
A basic meal should include about 70% grains, 30% is a mixture of vegetables, fruits, and meat. Grains contain Yang energy which Taoists believe to supply nutrients and boost vitality.

The Quan Zhen forbids garlic, chives, coriander, etc. from cooking since it affects the flow of energy and Harmony.

The Zhen Yi allows all things without restriction but advises cooked food over raw.

Ingredients must be mature and ripe without artificial enhancers.

2. Vegetables over meat
Instead of meat which is eaten in small quantities, vegetables are preferred. The meat encouraged for consumption is fresh and quality. These animals are prohibited for all who practice Taoism:

- Buffalo - are selfless and hard-working animals that consume grass and secrete milk. So, they are respected and seen as sacred.
- Mullet - this fish is sacrificial, exhibits genuine love and respect for its mother since the babies offer themselves to be eaten by their mother.
- Crane - faithful to one partner throughout their lifetime.
- Dig - loyal and of great help to man.

3. A little flavored and balanced meal
The harmony between your body and spirit is attainable when you also pay attention to diet. The five significant flavors from the Earth's element are connected to diet in Tao:

- Excess sour hurts spleen, Sourness for Wood
- Excess sweetness hurts kidney, Sweetness for the Earth
- Excess bitter hurts lung, Bitterness for Fire
- Excess spice hurts liver, Spiciness for Metal
- Excess salt hurts heart, Saltiness for Water

Balance in the Way cuts across all aspects of life. There should be no need for a flavor to overshadow another in a meal. All tastes should be in the right proportion for harmony.

Food like whole grains, vegetables (consumed steamed or fried), and a small proportion of meat is the ideal diet for Taoists. Fishes like salmon with high Yin components should be avoided while others are eaten once a week, red and blue hearts are prohibited, and games are consumed in moderate forms.

What do you eat?
To enjoy longevity, eating wisely is non-negotiable. Make sure to consume natural foods to boost your body's balance and functioning for optimum results. Healthy food should be consumed to preserve our bodies.

What is healthy food?
These are animals, minerals, and plants consumed or externally used on the body to hinder and provide healing for ailments by restoring the energy flow and making quality nutrients available for body (cells and tissues) regeneration.

Disobedience to nature's provision causes Bing; abnormal health in man. Diseases have been categorized into Air, Water, and Blood Dis-ease. This helps to understand the causes of these problems and tackle them at once.

4. The ideal medicine is food
The effect of food on our minds and physique is great. A lot of us eat thrice daily yet, we make the wrong food choices and end up consuming toxins. After a prolonged period, it accumulates and causes health challenges. Taoist advocates know how to use meals and herbs in balancing and providing nourishment to the body and mind to the extent that the body becomes light

and our consciousness expands. Taoists treat diseases with the food eaten daily, for instance, Yang deficiency is cured using mutton soup, Chinese angelica, and ginger; endemic goiter is cured with seaweed medicinal wine while night blindness is cured pork liver.

5. Don't fill your stomach

It implies two things: eat till about 80% satisfaction. Do not fill your stomach. Also, avoid or eat little meat/oily food. Tai Ping Jing states that eating enough is vital. These days, most of us pay attention to the energy we get from food regardless of the energy our body will require to break down the meal. When the food is complex, it will take more energy to break down. Overloading our stomach with food keeps it active in doing work. This will shorten your lifespan and a belly filled till it's brim will hinder the flow of energy. Eating less makes your heart open and doing otherwise invites diseases.

Guidelines for the major meals of the day
We are advised to eat based on the energy shift from yin-yang daily, that is, having a proper and full course breakfast but less when noontime is past. Dinner should even be less than lunch because as the body's yang reduces, digestion does likewise.

Drink when thirsty; Eat when hungry. You are what you eat, digest, and cannot digest. When there is food in your system and you eat, it is as good as useless. Your body cannot make use of it because it is blocked. It either gets excreted or remains as toxic substances in the body. Drinking water when you are not thirsty leaves much work for your kidneys and may not be expelled. Eating late-night meals is bad rather, get a healthy snack and do not fill your stomach. It is easier to get a good night's sleep with your body at rest.

6. Pay attention to your body
It is better for you to pay attention to your body than its senses or nutritional advice. Lao Tzu urges us to know what our body needs both intrinsically and extrinsically. The fact that it looks attractive, tastes amazing, or is advised by the doctor does not mean it is good for you. What is good for the goose may not be good for the gander.

How to treat your body to aid digestion:
- Let your mood be happy when you eat: play some good tunes as you eat for your spleen and digestive process. Fix your mind on chewing, talk less, or do not at all.
- When you are served a meal of different temperatures, begin with the hot meal, next is warm, last the cold meal.
- After each meal, make sure to rinse or brush your mouth.
  - Mouth washing with tea removes bacteria and freshens breath.
  - Mouth wash with warm water is preferable after a hot meal.
  - Mouth wash with cold water for a cold meal.
- Massaging the stomach to take out bad energy from food consumed is popular among Taoists. Digestion is aided by massages and walks. However, serious physical activities are not allowed after meals.

Drinks

A major part of our body is formed by water. Taking healthy and living water is important to health. Water is not just in the volume or mineral constituents instead, it is the amount of life contained in it. Taoist believes in live water because it is easily absorbed by the water. Unfortunately, we do not have access to live water hence, tap or bottled water is more consumed except citizens of Switzerland and Norway. Water from natural sources like; rivers, springs, mountains, lakes should be taken if possible (it has more life/essence compared to bottled water).

Drinking about 8 cups or more of water daily is not something Taoist believe in. Find the right quantity your body needs and make that the standard for you. Average consumption of teas is preferable to living water. Why? It purifies the mind and is an accurate antidote for the body. A little bit of alcohol is permitted in some Taoist ancestry; it supports the flow of energy, herbal absorption, skin nourishment, and blood circulation. Consuming large quantities of alcohol destroys the kidneys and liver since they function as detoxification.

Bigu/Pigu Fasting

The Shen Nong Bible is also a Taoist classic which states that individuals who consume grains are full of wisdom hence, the Qi will make them live forever.

Bi: not to eat, Gu: grains translated no to grains. Taoists hold a belief that consuming grains hinder them from getting enlightened. It is a process of switching off the body's Yang and turning on the Yin. The brain functions uniquely at that state, the physical and spiritual energy are well harnessed, stress is reduced, there is a greater sense of enlightenment and connection. Bigu is in two forms:

- Abstaining from food and consuming Qi (Qigong professionals)
- Taking herbal mixtures without grain consumption

Bigu is a means of detoxification highly esteemed by Taoists. On a final note, maintaining diets is a personal goal and business. There is no food that is bad or good. Just as advised by Taoists, know yourself and create the standard you would follow. No two persons are the same and Tao also taught that it is good we accept ourselves. Do not feel discouraged if one person has been keeping up with his dietary changes or yielding results. Go at your pace because your immunity and body metabolic level differ from others; some are fast, others slow. These summarized habitual patterns should be at the tip of your fingers:

1. Have a natural attitude and flow with nature
2. Eat proper and balanced energy meals
3. Focus on your body's language
4. Keep fit, exercise regularly
5. Have a positive outlook
6. Engage in a spiritual activity
7. Practice!

A healthy body and total wellness cannot be achievable if we do not consciously work at it, and there's no better time to start than now. As long as you're flowing with nature, you are good on the Way.

Part II

THE SPIRIT

Chapter One

WHAT IS THE HUMAN SPIRIT?

The word spirit comes from the Latin spiritus (derived from spirare, "to blow") which means "breath, air." It could also mean "to inspire" (lat. Inspirare) and "to expire" (lat. Expirare). "Spirit," or spiritus, is also the translation of the Greek pneuma and the Hebrew ruach.

The word "spirit" could be given to anything that is very subtle and very active, so we find it in expressions of the old chemistry like spirit of wine (alcohol) or spirit of salt (hydrochloric acid).

The spirit can also refer to the principle of life or to the individual soul. We no longer meet this use, taken up by Leibniz, except in theological or even mystical discourses.

"Reasonable spirits or souls" are "images of the Divinity, or of the very Author of nature; so that the Spirits are able to enter into a kind of Society with God."

In contemporary philosophical language, "spirit" can be opposed to different notions:

- Opposed to matter, with a distinction between thought and the object of thought, matter; with analogies with subjective/objective or uniqueness/multitude in certain relationships;
- Opposed to nature for example in the freedom/necessity distinction;
- Opposed to the flesh and the instinct of animal life, we find here a meaning close to that of Reason:

"The flesh desires contrary to those of the spirit, and the spirit desires contrary to those of the flesh."

The Spirit in the religions

- *Spirit in Christianity*
  In his first epistle to the Thessalonians , Paul of Tarsus prays that our "whole being, spirit, soul and body" will be kept blameless at the Coming of the Lord (1Th 5:23).

The Catholic Church teaches that the distinction between soul and spirit does not introduce a duality into the soul. In the 9th century, during the Fourth Council of Constantinople in 869, there was a controversy over the relationship between soul and body. The 11th canon of this council affirmed the uniqueness of the soul.

It is the 9th century that the distinction is formalized between the soul and spirit. The spirit being traditionally associated with the thought and the soul with the feeling, it was previously considered that man could have a multiple nature (body, soul and spirit). The Christianity asserted the contrary, the unity of the human person (a body and soul) by denying the existence of the spirit, because it coincides with the soul:

"The unity of soul and body is so deep that one must regard the soul as the form of the body; that is to say, it is thanks to the spiritual soul that the body made up of matter is a human and living body; mind and matter, in man, are not two natures united, but rather their union forms a single nature."

The Roman Catholic Church therefore sought to deepen the meaning of the terms, which was not without controversy between the Church of Rome and the Churches of the East. In the catechism of the Catholic Church, the notion of soul is attached to an individual (unity of the human person and of the soul), while the spirit is also considered from a collective angle:

"The sacred heritage of faith (depositum fidei), contained in Holy Tradition and in Sacred Scripture, was entrusted by the apostles to the whole Church. By attaching themselves to Him, the whole holy people united to their pastors remain assiduously faithful to the teaching of the apostles and to fraternal communion, to the breaking of bread and to prayers, so that, in the maintenance, the practice and the confession of the faith transmitted, settled between pastors and faithful, a singular unity of spirit."

This is particularly well revealed in the introduction to the encyclical Fides et ratio:

"Faith and reason are like the two wings which allow the human spirit to rise towards the contemplation of the truth. It is God who put in the heart of man the desire to know the truth and, in the end, to know Him himself so that, knowing Him and loving Him, he can attain the full truth about himself."

The word "spirit", with a lower case (therefore that of man), appears very often in this encyclical, while the word "soul" appears only five times.

The word Spirit written with a capital letter, or appearing in the names Spirit of truth, Spirit of adoption... (always with a capital letter) designates the Holy Spirit.

• *The spirit in the Kabbalah*
  Jewish mysticism, from the 11th century, believes that man has, besides the physical body, many souls. The Jewish neo-Platonists Abraham ibn Ezra (c. 1150) and Abraham bar Hiyya Hanassi distinguish three parts: nêfesh, ru'ah, neshamah; kabbalists add hayyah, yehidah. The five names of the soul are, in ascending order: the nêfesh ("vitality", "bodily double"), the ru'ah ("breath", the "personality", the anima), the neshamah ("the divine perfume", "higher soul", "divine spark", "spiritus"), the hayyah ("Divine life", equivalent of Buddhi) and the yehidah ("union", "oneness", indivisible principle of individuality). If we group together in an acronym the initials of each of these terms we obtain the word naran-hai, ("Living Fire"). This is the doctrine of the Kabbalist Isaac Louria, around 1570, at Safed.

• *The spirit in Buddhism*
  The Buddhism denies the existence of the soul (considers as an illusion), and emphasizes the interdependence between the deep body and mind. The individual is considered there as a set of aggregates, the first of which is the body, accompanied by four other concepts that can be linked

to the notion of spirit: sensations, perceptions, volitional formations and consciousness.

These aggregates are impermanent and interdependent processes, not immutable objects. The mind is linked to the body and becomes truly independent of it only in the sublimated states of meditation which are the dhyānas in view of nirvāna.

The mind is considered, not as a "ghost in the machine" of the body, but as a sixth sense (manas) in addition to the five senses usually recognized. Buddhism is neither spiritualist nor materialist: the mind is not an eternal entity, but it is not an epiphenomenon of matter either. The brain is only a kind of "terminal" which operates the interface between the mind (immaterial) and the world of the five senses (material). Experiences of altered states of consciousness, common in advanced meditators, seem to confirm this view.

Ajahn Brahm explains:
"The sixth sense, the mind, is independent of the other five senses. In particular, it is independent of the brain. If there was a brain transplant between you and me, you took my brain and I took yours, I would still be Ajahn Brahm and you would still be you."

The Dalai Lama expresses a similar opinion:
"The highest level [of consciousness] escapes material support. Consciousness is independent of physical particles."

The fundamental functioning of the mind and its conditioning in saṃsāra are described by the causal chain of conditioned co-production. Some schools, like the Cittamātra school, teach an unconscious aspect of the mind, Ālayavijñāna.

The spirit in philosophies

- *Classical Western Philosophy*
  In the 17th century, Descartes separates the body from the mind (he identifies the soul) in a dualism: the body is an extended substance and is the mechanical (hence the theory of animal-machine) while the soul is a thinking substance. When passive, the mind is intellect; as an asset, it is will. The unity of the two remains a thorny problem, and Descartes sees the pineal gland as the place of communication between the two.

More simply, Descartes breaks down the mind into three components: thought, imagination and memory.

Conversely, the proponents of philosophical materialism refuse the existence of an immaterial principle and the mind is conceived as the manifestation of physiological phenomena governed by the laws of physics: "the brain secretes thought as the liver secretes bile " (Pierre-Jean-Georges Cabanis, 1802).

Philosophy of contemporary spirit
The generalization of the monistic naturalistic paradigm in the sciences of the mind, known today as the cognitive sciences, often leads today to putting between the brain and the mind the same type of relationship as between the material ("Hardware") and software ("software") in IT.

This thesis known as the brain-computer metaphor also knows its adversaries, those who refuse to see in the mind only an epiphenomenon of neurobiology, opposing the optimism of those for whom, the field of "this which remains to be explained in the functioning of the mind" is finished and is shrinking from year to year.

Spiritualist philosophy
The spiritualism is defined as a spiritual philosophy and grant an essential place to the concept of mind. For this doctrine, the spirit is the intelligent principle of the universe, whose true nature remains to be discovered.

In the sense of the spiritualist doctrine, the Spirits are the intelligent beings of creation, which inhabit the universe outside the material world, and which constitute the invisible world. They are not beings of a particular creation, but the souls of those who have lived on earth or in other spheres, and who have left their bodily envelope.

The spirit in the sciences

By etymology, psychology is the science of the mind. But faced with the religious and mystical connotations of the word, scientific discourse has preferred to use more neutral terms such as those of mental faculties or processes or even psyche (especially in approaches inspired by psychoanalysis) or cognition. In contemporary cognitive science, the term cognition does not only refer to the faculties of knowledge and intelligence (of thought) but to all the psychological processes at work in the human (and non-human) mind, including perception, motivation, decision or emotions.

Indeed, it is found in 1983 used in the translation of the book of the philosopher Jerry Fodor, The Modularity of Mind and in the following expressions:

The philosophy of mind, the branch of contemporary philosophy which focuses on the problems of the concepts of mind, mental states, consciousness, etc.

The theory of mind is this psychological faculty in a very small number of animal species, or, according to some researchers, specific to humans that allows an individual to understand the mental states (beliefs and intentions) another individual.

The "Society of the Mind" is the title of a book by Marvin Minsky in which he proposes to analyze human cognition as a holistic phenomenon, emerging from the interaction of a very large number of agents themselves unintelligent.

The notion of ecology of the mind was developed by anthropologist Gregory Bateson in his book Ecology of the Mind and can be compared with that of ecology of consciousness by neuropsychologist Gerald Edelman.

Chapter Two

THE ROLE OF THE SPIRIT IN THE (PHYSICAL) WORLD

The term spirit can be applied, according to the oldest interpretations, to living beings in general (plants and animals) as its constitutive principle. According to some interpretations, such as Aristotle's, the soul would incorporate the vital principle or internal essence of each of these living beings, thanks to which they have a certain identity, which cannot be explained from the material reality of its parts.

The term is also used in a more particular sense if it refers to human beings; in this second case, according to many religious and philosophical traditions, the soul would be the spiritual component of human beings.

In the course of history, the concept of the spirit goes through various attempts at explanation: from the dualism of philosophical idealism and gnosis to the existentialist interpretation of a whole with two specific aspects that are: the material and the immaterial.

For the Christian religion, man consists of three parts that are: body (the physical), soul (related to the emotional) and spirit (related to the spiritual). According to the Christian tradition, the spirit is one of the aspects of the human being that unifies him as an individual and "launches" him into activities that go beyond the material. Thanks to the soul, the human being has free instincts, feelings, emotions, thoughts and decisions, and can return to himself (self-consciousness).

Although it is not very frequent, the term "soul" can also be used referring to any human being as a whole, ignoring the religious or philosophical meaning, as in the expressions "there is not even a soul" or "city of 40,000 souls."

The soul in western philosophy

- *Greek philosophy*
  Plato considered the spirit as the most important dimension of the human being. Sometimes he speaks of her as if she were imprisoned in a body, although this idea is borrowed from Orphism.

According to the Timaeus, the spirit was composed of the identical and the diverse, a substance that the demiurge used to create the cosmic soul and the other stars; Furthermore, the lower gods created two mortal spirit: the passionate, which resides in the thorax, and the appetitive, which resides in the abdomen. Above both would be the rational soul, which would find its place in the head.

Something similar is narrated in the Phaedrus, where the myth of the winged horses is exposed: the charioteer is the rational spirit, the white horse represents the passionate part and the black the part of the appetites (always rebellious). The charioteer's task is to keep the black horse at the same gallop as the white. In the Phaedo, the spirit is seen as a substance that seeks to detach itself from the limits and conflicts that arise from its union with the body, and that will be able to live fully after the moment of death; This dialogue offers various arguments that seek to prove her immortality.

Aristotle defined the Psyche as "a specific form of a natural body that potentially has life, (From Anima, 412 a20)." He also understands it as "the essence of such a type of body" (412b10). The form or essence is what makes an entity what it is. By this we understand that the soul is what defines a natural body. For example, if the ear were an animal, its spirit would be listening and its matter the ear's own organ. An ear that did not have the function of hearing would be an ear only for words. In this case, the spirit configures matter in an organized natural body.

Thus a substantial unit (composed of matter and form) is formed. Spirit and body are not separable in the living being.

The spirit is also defined by the stagirite as "the first entelechy of a natural body that potentially has life" (412a26). This indicates that the spirit is entelechy or first act of the living body and soul and body are united simultaneously. But since the spirit is the act, it can be said that it has priority over the body. It is first not in time, but in importance. It is the first action from which the faculties and powers of the living being arise.

Aristotle points out, finally, that there could be operations of the soul that did not depend on anybody.

The dualistic vision that emerges from Platonism distorts reality and the consequences come to a disregard for physical realities, the human body and sexuality, among other things. The spirit is imagined as something independent, part of the divine and of the good, like a white sheet stuck in a poor material envelope from which it is urgent to free itself.

However, Aristotelian monism allows us to understand the human being as a unit made up of body and soul, giving the body just value by not understanding it as the prison of the soul (as Plato did), but as an essential part of what man is.

Thomas Aquinas
With Thomas Aquinas, anthropological reflection (explanation of what the human being is) takes a more realistic turn. Drawing on Aristotle more than Plato, Thomas Aquinas speaks of principles, no longer of opposite realities. For Aristotle, all beings in the physical world have matter (which is pure indeterminacy) and a substantial form (which is the determinative principle).

These two realities are inseparable, so they have no independent existence. We would say that these are two "aspects" of the same reality. Thomas Aquinas describes the human being as material on the one hand (his body) and not material on the other (his spirit). The human being is immersed in the material and obeys its basic laws of space and time. At the same time, it shows that it is not material at all, being able to go beyond space and time with its reason: planning the future or arranging the arrangements on an existing space in its daily life.

Example: I can prepare an agenda for tomorrow and conceptualize what the dining room of the house will be like without having to be present in that dining room.

Spirit and body become co-principles in the explanation of what the human being is like. The human being is fully bodily but has something of his own that allows him to go beyond the bodily: his spiritual soul. However, it is the soul that has the being in the first place, while the body exists as united to the soul.

Later western thought
Western thought fell on the dualism between body and spirit:

Descartes defines soul as a thinking thing as opposed to an "extensive" thing (res cogitans versus res Amplia).

a. Baruch Spinoza speaks of the soul as an attribute and mode of the divine substance.
b. Leibniz calls it a monad closed in on itself.
c. Theodor Lessing, as infinite aspiration.
d. Kant describes it as the impossibility of learning the absolute.
e. Fichte, how to know and action.
f. Hegel says that the soul is the self-development of the idea.
g. Friedrich Schelling defines it as a mystical power.
h. Nietzsche, invention and imaginary entity of the common people, that helps to strengthen the beliefs of the existence of a god or, more specifically, of "God".

i. Freud, as the difference between the "I" and the "super-me".

j. Jaspers defines it as "existentiality".

k. Ernst Bloch, as the original realization of the future.

In the Judeo-Christian tradition
According to the Judeo-Christian religious tradition, the spirit is the main identifying quality of movement in living matter, making it non-moving (inert) to moving, independent of the displacement of others.

According to the biblical records, in Genesis (Genesis 1: 20-28) it says:

- 20, God said: "Let the waters be filled with a multitude of living beings and let birds fly over the earth, through the firmament of the sky."

- 21, God created the great sea monsters, the various kinds of living beings that fill the waters by gliding in them, and all species of animals with wings. And God saw that this was good.

- 22, Then he blessed them, saying: "Be fruitful and multiply; fill the waters of the seas and let the birds multiply on the earth.

- 23, Thus there was an evening and a morning: this was the fifth day.

- 24, God said, "May the earth produce all kinds of living things: cattle, reptiles, and wild animals of all kinds." And so it happened.

- 25, God made the various kinds of animals of the field, the various kinds of cattle, and all the reptiles of the earth, whatever their species. And God saw that this was good.

- 26, God said, "Let us make man in our image, after our likeness; and that the fish of the sea and the birds of the sky, the cattle, the beasts of the earth and all the animals that crawl on the ground are subject to it.

- 27, And God created man in his image; He created him in the image of God, He created them male and female.

- 28, And he blessed them, saying: "Be fruitful, multiply, fill the earth and subdue it; dominate the fish of the sea, the birds of the sky and all the living beings that move on the earth.

The term also appears in the anthropological vision of numerous cultural and religious groups. In the modern era, the term "soul" is used more frequently in religious contexts

The spirit, in Christian theology
Christian theology, mainly German Protestant theology, is inspired by Idealism (current based on ideas) and comes to conceive of the soul as only "subjectivity". This same Idealism influences through Descartes the thought of some Catholic currents. Indeed, Descartes, by stating "I think, therefore I am", encloses philosophical reflection in the world of ideas. He is considered the father of idealism.

The philosophers cited in the previous paragraph are, for the most part, "idealistic" philosophers.

The philosophical realism gave birth to both the empiricism and the Marxism as existentialist philosophy (existentialism) and Christian existentialism (Gabriel Marcel, personalism of Mounier).

In the Bible

In the Bible, the word "soul" is given as a translation of the Hebrew word (ne '• phesch [נֶפֶשׁ]) and the Greek word (psy • khe'). From the use of the word in the Bible, it is clear that the soul is the person or animal itself referred to by the term, or the life that the person or animal enjoys.

The rúaj, which is "wind", "spirit" in Hebrew, in relation to anthropology is the 'breath [of life]', breath of the divinity itself: when Yahweh breathed on man his breath of life (Genesis 2: 7), it became a living being. Man lives while Yahweh does not withdraw his reach, (Job 27.3). The term strongly marks the relationship between creature and creator, her absolute dependence on Him.

The Ruach receives other meanings in the Bible according to the contexts. The nephesh (נפש) means "throat", "jaws" (2 Samuel 16:14), "one who breathes" (Job 41:13, 20, 21). Néfesch comes from a root that means "to breathe", and in a literal sense it could be translated as "a respirator."

Exactly the same Hebrew expression that is used for the animal creation, namely, néfesch jaiyah (living soul), is applied to Adam when it is said that after God formed man from the dust of the ground and blew into his nostrils the breath of life, "man became a living soul" (Ge 2:7).

In the instructions that God gave to man after creating him, he used the term "nefesch" again to refer to the animal creation: in which there is life as a soul [literally, in which there is a living soul (nephesh)] "(Genesis 1:30).

Sometimes the word né • fesch is used to express the desire of the individual, which fulfills him and then pushes him to achieve his goal. Proverbs 13:2 says of those who treat treacherously that 'their very soul is violence,' that is, they are staunch supporters of violence, and actually become violence personified - so it has to do with interaction as well. between the mind and active personality of an individual, "life" (1 Samuel 26:21).

Also, the Genesis 9: 4 record says that the blood is Alma and Leviticus 17:11 says that the blood is the soul, because each living cell that makes up the blood is capable of moving in itself, differentiating animal beings from plants, which do not have blood or cells related to it; the blood, whose cellular movement allows the convolution of respiration, shows its distinctive characteristic of Animal Life. The word néfesch (נפש) appears a total of 754 times in the Hebrew Scriptures (Genesis to Malachi) and its Greek equivalent psykhḗ (ψυχή) 105 times in the Greek Scriptures(Matthew to Revelation) and is never associated with the immortality that some religious, philosophical or other currents give it. But most notably, there are hundreds of biblical texts that associate it with death; in fact, there are 13 texts where it is mentioned as "dead néfesch" (dead soul).

Also, they do not have to do psykhḗ (ψυχή) and the Latin word anima (words that are related to the Spanish term «animal," making the expression « rational animal « logical for the human being) with the word spirit (gr. pneuma).

So, the spirit is defined by inseparable interaction of three movements in living matter that make it up: Mind/Heart (conscious-unconscious psychological principle of the Self [pneumatic movement]), Blood (principle of the animal or carnal body [lymphatic movement]) and Life (principle of activity-habit [dynamic movement]).

Without these three, the soul is dead. From this interpretation arises the importance of valuing both the human spirit and that of a beast. Strengthening the ethical evaluation from the most sensitive part of the soul (mind/ heart) until the toughest part of it (life).

The basár (flesh) is a concept that is not opposed to rúaj (breath) but they are juxtaposed. An acceptable translation would be "my person", which can be touched, experienced. When Paul says: "Your bodies are the temple of the Spirit (in gr. Pneuma) ... (1 Cor 6,19)" or "You are the temple ... (1 Cor, 3-17)" he highlights the aspect experienceable of the concept.

The Catholic Magisterium
The dogmatic definitions of the Magisterium of the Catholic Church deal mainly with the relationships between soul and body. The main:

- The man has a spirit
- The spirit exists in each man as individually distinct and is immortal in this individual diversity.
- The spirit is a corporeal form by itself.

From Pope John XXII:

a. The spirit can have the full vision of God, only after death. The spirit is created and infused immediately by God at the moment of conception.
b. The spirit does not belong to the divine substance.
c. The spirit does not lead a pre-corporeal existence.
d. The spirit does not have a material origin.
e. She constitutes the vital principle of man.
f. It is superior to the body.
g. Your spirituality can be demonstrated.

The Second Vatican Council goes beyond the soul-body scheme and speaks of the person. "Man is one body and soul, and in his interiority transcends all things …"

Pope John Paul II in a Sunday locution, published in L'Osservatore Romano (01/14/1990), said that "animals possess a vital breath received from God", quoting Psalms 103 and 104, being recognized, therefore, the 'sensitive soul' (Greek 'pneuma', breath, air), without forgetting that the word 'animal' comes from the Latin 'anima' (spirit). "Animals have a spirit and human beings must love and feel solidarity with our younger brothers."

Iconography
The early Christians represented in their monuments the human soul free from the shackles of the flesh and addressing the heavenly homeland by means of the following symbolic figures:

a. A horse running as if to get the prize in the circus games.
b. A ship sailing with unfolded sails towards a lighthouse or arriving at the port.

c. A lamb or a sheep alone or restored to the flock by the Good Shepherd.

d. A dove sometimes flying, sometimes next to an empty glass, an image of the body abandoned by the spirit and other times perched in a flowery garden, representing Paradise.

e. A woman emerging from an inanimate body.

The spirit in other cultures
Oriental meditation for the purification of the soul.

In other cultures such as Asian, African, and American, we find a spirit concept analogously similar to the concept developed by the religions of the Judeo-Christian group (including Islam) and European philosophy.

The spirit from the Vedic or Veda point of view, is The Self (Atman), which by nature is eternal (without birth or death or without beginning or end) of substance different from that of the physical body and which has its own consciousness.

From this perspective, material science, or that which studies physical or material phenomena, is limited because it cannot study spiritual phenomena since its nature is different from physical.

Spirit in Ancient Egypt
The human being, according to the ancient Egyptians, has seven degrees in his personality:

a. "Ren", that is "the name", being able to remain existing according to the care of a correct embalming.

b. "Sechem" is the energy, the power, the light of the deceased.

c. "Aj" is the unification of "Ka" and "Ba", in view of a return to existence.

d. "Ba", what makes an individual being what it is; it also applies to inanimate things. It is the closest to the western concept of "Soul".

e. "Ka", the life force. Supported by food offerings to the deceased.

f. "Sheut" is the shadow of the person, represented by a completely black human figure.

g. "Seju" designates the physical remains of the person.

h. "Jat" is the carnal part of the person.

Buddhist beliefs

One of the three marks of existence, Anātman is the "Insubstantiality of things". Nowhere does the scripture speak of an intrinsic essence of being or something inner with which to connect. It is normal to confuse the "Ultimate Reality" of the mind which is the indestructible "Buddha Nature" like a diamond (Vajra Sattva); however, on a philosophical level that indestructible nature is the emptiness of things and is completely different from the concept of Atman, soul, Being, etc. Those concepts are considered to arise from the ego and confusion of the mind.

The Buddhism teaches that all things are changing in a constant state of flux. Everything is temporary and there is no something perennial. That applies to the entire cosmos and therefore to humanity itself. There is no permanent "I". Anātman expresses in essence the Buddhist idea of that continuous change.

The mistake of believing in a permanent "I" is the source of human conflicts and worldly desires. Attachment to the defects of cyclical existence, samsara, brings about rebirth.

When it comes to rebirth, in Buddhism, it is the ego and the manifestation of the confused mind, of the stream of consciousness. The concept of reincarnation is also used, although it is not as correct as the previous one; however, there is no exact translation for the concept so far.

The Buddhism believes that there are three levels in the consciousness of the person: very subtle consciousness, which does not disintegrate in the incarnation-death, the subtle consciousness, which disappears with death and is a consciousness-asleep or non-consciousness, and gross conscience.

Hindu beliefs
The religions that speak about the spirit such as the Hindu, which arose from the Vedas, which are sacred texts for the Hindus, where they speak of life that there is a transmigration of the soul, that is called the wheel of samsara. Death is when the spirit passes from one body to another according to its actions or how it leads its life; This process of the soul was given changes and it became known as Dharma, which is the result of a good life or doing well and karma is everything that must necessarily live to learn from life so that in another life it can become better person.

Buddha, who to some extent has been considered one of the representatives of Hindu culture, says that to save the soul one must reach the state of nirvana, which is the highest state of harmony.

Meditation helps purify the soul and food is very important to achieve nirvana, since life is sacred. Nirvana is also achieved by having a life of holiness, for example, not committing impure acts that can affect the soul and learning to control vices and bad influences.

Iconology

The butterfly was among the ancients the emblem or image of the spirit. The artists of antiquity represented Plato with butterfly wings on his head, because he was the first Greek philosopher who dealt with the immortality of the spirit. An ancient fragment from Stosch's cabinet represents the meditation of a philosopher with a butterfly placed on a skull in front of which the philosopher is reflecting.

The purification of the soul by fire is expressed in a small sepulchral urn in the city of Mattei, through Love that has a butterfly in its hand to which a lit torch approache. A butterfly flying over the mouth of a comic mask seems to indicate that the wearer is alive or animated.

Sometimes Cupid is seen taking by the wings a butterfly that is crumbling, a symbol of the torments that love makes the hearts it dominates suffer.

Chapter Three

THE GOOD, THE BAD, AND THE SPIRIT

Don't get things twisted. Spirituality does not mean religiosity. Religions aim at strict beliefs (dogmas), following certain rules and sometimes even power games to control people, their members or even other people while spirituality is about the question of the meaning of life in a larger context.

Ultimately, nothing else is meant by the term esotericism. Of course there is a common intersection between religion and spirituality. Any positive form of religious orientation should be spiritual, but not every spiritual way of thinking and living is religious. That is infinitely important.

Spiritual vs. material existence

There are now two extremes: those who do not want to deal with spirituality and only think in terms of worldly parameters. The others who flatly reject worldly views and want to devote themselves exclusively to their spiritual existence. This form of duality is out of place. The society of the future will have to manage to integrate both aspects of its incarnated self into everyday life.

Why not live purely materially?
The properties that we want to develop further cannot be fully described rationally. If we still want to try: it is about the qualities of energies as modern quantum physics must grudgingly assume in order to be able to describe all properties of the behavior of elementary particles. Examples of these qualities are bliss, humility, lightning ideas, and ubiquitous love. In a purely material mindset, we will not experience these things and waste our incarnation.

Why not live purely spiritually?
We made a conscious decision for an incarnation. An incarnation is by definition tied to a material existence. This material formation may, can and should help us to further develop certain characteristics of ourselves in a way that we as purely spiritual beings would otherwise not be able to do. A denial of our material world is therefore not expedient for our spiritual existence.

How do we integrate a spiritual attitude into our everyday life?
We have all arrived very well in the purely worldly world. The question arises as to how we can integrate our natural spirituality into everyday life. To do this, we have to check what people have been doing wrong so far in order to prevent precisely that.

Human problems in everyday life
Unfortunately, people generally like to differentiate. It starts with the separation in work and personal life. A very misleading

distinction. If we mark out an area of our life in which we are not ourselves, but surrender to a world that deliberately exposes us to malaise as a means to an end (money), we purposefully create an environment that is not good for us.

Free and creative
It is important that we find the expression of our inner love in everything we do. However, this is about a basic form of love, different from the popular vernacular. It's about effortless kindness, compassion for everything that happens. The result is an opening of the heart towards wholeness (not only inward, not only outward). Dissolving negative beliefs is a symptom of this heart integration, an increase in vibration and the rejection of drug abuse.

Confidence and devotion develop, which serves everything that surrounds us - including our "work", if we let it become part of it and do what corresponds to our passion.

From matter to spirituality
Today's top-heavy people begin their journey by wanting to understand. The questions are "Who am I?", "Where do I come from?", "Who was I in my previous life?", and "Where should I go? " These questions are a good sign. The nature of creation is then explored with a changed view of nature and all incoming experiences examined with regard to their origin, content and purpose. Everything is questioned. Material reality is no longer seen as an origin, but as a symptom of a superordinate structure. One pursues such thoughts more intensely, the other more superficially.

Gradually, we are looking for what is hidden from the simple self. The everyday life of spirituality is characterized by the perception of unchangeable processes of worldly existence (seasons, sleep rhythms, metabolism, etc.). This perception is an important part of becoming aware. It is like slowly waking up from a sleep that has arisen from our personality, which has been programmed by various influences. This perception is considered the most basic form of meditation in Buddhism.

From the spiritual world towards matter
Just as we slowly (again) begin to be interested in the spiritual world, the openness to influences from this very spiritual world grows in our direction. We are not on our own while we want to contest our development. Strictly speaking, we have a whole team of spiritual helpers who we can ask for help. They do not serve to relieve us of our tasks. On the contrary, they will (at our former, specific request) do nothing that stands in the way of our learning task, ie our development.

However, assuming a sufficiently mature consciousness, they will be available to us with a multitude of answers to various questions of existence - because we already know all this, but we just weren't able to take it with us into this incarnation. Our higher self is ultimately more than our simple self, only "unfortunately" does not incarnate the higher self.

Spiritual helpers consist, for example, of our spirit guide who had incarnated himself once and who accompanies us throughout our entire incarnation. Another helper is our guardian angel, who is with us our entire soul life, never had to incarnate, but also does not protect us in the conventional sense (ie not our body), but ensures that we can cope with our learning tasks here. He ensures that our constantly changing circumstances meet our learning task.

It is amusing how our spirit guide alone supports us in some of the simplest everyday tasks, for example opening a can ("Be careful! Other side!"), or before opening someone else's refrigerator ("Slow down, something is about to fly towards you!"). We should accept this help. But we can also ask specific questions to which we may receive an answer that we will understand. If not, we can always ask for signs that we can understand.

The limits of personality

We can already see that the world is not perceived as a whole in the ego. All areas of life are perceived and described separately. At best we can explain how these supposedly separate aspects work together. All of this can be seen in the division of the sciences into physics, biology, psychology, etc. We separate everything.

At the same time, we still see ourselves exposed to high influences. Both are due to the same problem. Our ego manifestation enriches the need for energetic protection (click here) and positive boundaries, which on the one hand is important for one's own integrity in our current society, but on the other hand is also precisely part of the overarching problem that characterizes society.

In any case, it reinforces the fragmented perception in parts, away from the whole. A first step to serve both the development of society and oneself would be to reduce the speed with which we deal with this world through thinking, feeling and acting.

This will also do the area of our interpersonal relationships very well, and it will also allow our consciousness to mature through more honest, relaxed and easy acceptance of honest feedback from the partner.

Spirituality in everyday life; Enjoyment in the now
Life should become meditation. It starts with conscious breathing in every moment. We can also:

- Walk consciously
- Be more aware of your own movements
- Eat more consciously
  and so on.

It is of central importance to get to know yourself, to dissolve your own blockages, to experience your own hidden talents and abilities. All of this is possible from within, but can also be done through external aids - the "book of your life", for example, can help you to get to know your soul. However, the natural maturation of the empathic sense can only take place from within.

With everything that can be achieved in this material world, however, the golden goal is to always live in the here and now, no matter how difficult it is to keep. Otherwise we practice so much with cramped goals - that would be a really worthwhile one. If you want to choose the most direct route, you can try DMT. The experience with an ayahuasca potion comes very close to deep meditation. But generating the frequencies yourself is always the more sustainable way.

Ultimately, however, the question is, how do we still achieve what we have to do here on earth? After all, we don't want to develop a split personality? To live in the here and now is in apparent contradiction to the material existence in which one should live out one's abilities. But that's not a contradiction in terms. Planning and acting does not mean that you cannot enjoy the journey to your destination - and vice versa.

If we make regular friends, that means not just planning and chasing goals that we assume that our life will only begin afterwards, something exciting will happen. The result is a deep phase of cleaning up contaminated sites. Old emotional or mental blockages in the form of trauma or thought patterns, beliefs or automated actions that have become irrelevant slowly dissolve. Mindfulness sets in.

One comes to naturally being in the here and now. But not in the sense of intoxicating, lasting pleasure satisfaction, but in the sense of centered liveliness. We get to know a stream of life that goes from above into the head, through the entire body and into the feet. Our consciousness will increase exponentially. We are becoming clearer, more permeable, more sublime - and even more creative.

Sublime task completion
Increased awareness creates an inner calm in us, with which we do our tasks. We are considerate of ourselves and others, and thus, in a slower way, we may even manage more than before. In any case, we are less carried away and less lost in frequent courses of action and activities. Thus, we are also less charged with external energies, which makes energetic protection just as less necessary as the processing of stressful everyday experiences through the psyche (for example during sleep). If

you are part of the described stream of life, you are on the one hand more part of everything, but at the same time the whole is also much more in us, which not least also increases our (real) self-confidence.

People are very fond of, and extremely quickly, differentiating between "good" and "bad". He can classify good people and good deeds just as quickly as he can classify bad people and bad deeds. Society has trained itself to use thought patterns that are predefined by supposedly clear moral concepts and kept stable by literature, film and media reports. This article is intended to critically examine the perspectives on "good" and "bad" and end in a conclusion as to whether and when these attributes make sense. In order to approach these questions, each reader should be as open in mind and heart as humanly possible.

Evil from the point of view of society

Let's first clarify what the vernacular thinks is good and bad. Good people obey moral standards. You have a conscience and you use it. But this is where the differences begin. What is considered moral and what is not is subjective. One perceives a white lie with the boss as a necessary means to get ahead in life, the other perceives it as very reprehensible. So the first problem is already the basis of what we see as a reference for good or bad behavior.

The second problem is valuation. If we assume clearly defined foundations for moral behavior, if we equate morality with legal texts, the question still remains of how I evaluate a situation against this (for the moment, uniform) basis. Let's make a rough distinction here between the rational and the emotional view.

The rationally thinking person judges coolly and on the basis of facts, weights the available information about the behavior of a person perhaps using a key along criteria and finally comes to a result: 92.5% moral. The heart-centered person may take into account the particular circumstances of the person(s) involved in the particular situation. It does not come to a value, but to a tendency, a qualitative demarcation. So he could only compare two differently acting individuals against our moral basis from the beginning: Person A acted more morally.

For example, is it good or bad to help a homeless person? The rational person can argue: with a donation I promote the laziness of the individual, and thus the fact that people sabotage society. The heart man can argue: it is a different being, it may not be to blame for what happened to it, it is my duty to help it. Who's Right - Nobody? both? And finally: who should finally assess this and make a decision? Only society as a whole can do that.

No matter from which direction we come, whether mind or heart have priority, or we try to incorporate both as best as possible (subjectively), there will be no really stable evaluation scheme, so no moral police makes sense. Even with actually uniform requirements, the laws, there is still a lot of leeway for legal disputes depending on the situation and circumstances, why should it look better with far more subjective things such as human morality.

Nevertheless, people will always agree on very specific points: if I help an old woman across the street, it is "good", if I kill someone else, it is "bad". Is that generally true, or are we still making it too easy for ourselves here?

Evil in Humans: Society vs. the view of psychology
No psychologist will say that murder is a defensible thing. Also, no psychologist will say that certain women should not be helped across the street. But if we take a look at how the topic of criminal therapy is dealt with, one discovers, among other things, the following, very consistent trace of prejudice along the supposedly enlightened society:

- "Therapists only see the good in people, even if that doesn't exist"
- "As soon as someone feigns repentance, he is pardoned"
- "Therapy for offenders is just pointless pampering"
  Society is certain: good people don't kill anyone, only bad people do that, and they should be locked away or killed.
- *Evil people as an incarnation of horror?*

First of all, one could immediately object to the fact that if we keep criminals locked up or even killed, we as a society can never learn what they did and how it could be prevented from other potential perpetrators in the future. However, this already implies an understanding of what many people lack: people are not simply born bad, they are made to commit acts that the majority of society considers evil through certain abuses that are perpetrated on them.

There is absolutely no question that certain acts should not have any excuse. Nevertheless, psychology sees each person as the sum of different character building blocks that are formed by various factors. Certain intensities and constellations of these characteristics make a person more likely to commit "bad" deeds than others in certain situations.

From this, it can immediately be deduced that many people who could actually be potentially very dangerous simply never experience a situation in which they have to commit a crime. Example: Husbands are killed by their wives far less often than in the past, since divorces now result in an equal separation of property. Many potential murderers simply no longer have to commit murder - due to a lack of social "necessity."

Other people, on the other hand, may even have less potential to become criminals, but have a sufficiently strong situation that they trigger certain "bad" actions. Fortunately, many others have neither the necessary building blocks in the necessary mature form nor a situation in which they could prove their "malevolence."

So we are slowly starting to see that psychology deals much more sensibly with the subject of "good" and "bad". It simply excludes these terms as attributes of a person. A kind of modular principle prevails here, an attribution that provides a certain potential for certain actions, the execution of which requires a trigger.

Whether the respective action is then classified as less good or even as malicious is up to (a) the viewer and (b) the applicable assessment basis. We should ask ourselves whether we ourselves don't do something once a week that others would classify as "bad" in a certain way, but which we ourselves can excellently justify. Just as it happens all the time around us in small, hopefully insignificant situations around us, it can also be the case on a large scale.

Psychology sees not only the symptoms of an action, but judiciously to their cause, of course, with the aim of repairing act on these (and not about sweeping assumption that without exception every person would be treatable, and cannot be more today so easily deceive as before). Above all, however, it does not expose an action to an ad hoc vote in the form of "good" and "bad."

Curse and blessing of reason and the question of justice
The perspective of psychology is very positive here and on the one hand should be anchored much more deeply in society. This would make the topic of offender therapy much more mature and, last but not least, simplify the work of psychologists. The social benefit is ultimately more than obvious: if we learn to understand, we can learn to treat, and if we learn to treat, we can practice prevention. Initiatives like "Don't become a perpetrator" consist of the results of psychotherapeutic research.

But you quickly make a jump here. You might think to yourself that if there is no such thing as good and bad, then there is no real justice either, right? If people simply perform certain actions, each of which is a consequence of their legacy plus the triggering situation, everything is subject to chaos, right? The idea of a god or the like would also be off the table or he would be pretty disinterested or sadistic.

Here we come up against the limits of pure reason. As nice as it is not to be able to easily classify "good" and "bad", "justice" is still conceivable here on a completely different level.

The view of spirituality

A question that psychology does not ask itself in any way - and that is certainly not its task - is that of the origin of the contaminated sites. This is not intended to mean the influence of one person on another, for example a pedophile educator, whose victim later becomes the perpetrator himself. What is meant is why a soul gets into exactly such a situation in which it is exposed to such an educator.

When we talk about karma, it is important that we discuss legacy assumption. Contaminated territories are not tied to physical life. In a previous life we made certain experiences, but also made certain "free" decisions, which on the one hand expanded our own treasure trove of experiences and on the other hand also had an impact on other people/souls.

We are allowed to experience the consequence of this influence, assuming no honest repentance based on understanding/ empathy, at the latest in a subsequent incarnation, which we indirectly choose. This is how the topic of justice can also be described: from a purely psychological point of view, it is not fair if a person falls victim to another person just because they call certain circuits their own, no matter how well they can be explained psychologically.

From a spiritual point of view, however, we can rely on the fact that the big picture has a meaning and that there is - outside of the closed incarnations - a generally applicable justice. Of course, this initially eludes our understanding. However, there is evidence in the literature that raped women have been regressed to see how they molested other women in a previous life as a man.

Just as psychology does not want to find an excuse for the perpetrators' decisions, spirituality should not be understood at this point as a free ticket for negative actions, this does not have to be emphasized. Only one view should be motivated, which makes justice explainable in the absence of objectively definable malice.

But what about the terms "good" and "bad" themselves? What is exciting here is that, based on this superordinate view, benevolent (light) energetic influences can very well prevail - and always when they specifically neutralize lower - frequency areas. In terms of a generally valid origin of certain energetic patterns that influence everything that is, we can of course speak of "good" and "bad". Yes, there is a devil, demons, goblins and more (if we want to call these beings that). There is also black magic and "bad" witches - people who use their conscious connection for malicious purposes.

Evil as a means to an end
But here on earth we are always exposed to both influences: the positive and the negative, and it is up to us to develop towards the light. It is important to bristle with the negative influences, and this is exactly why these low-frequency influences are so important. "Lucifer" means Bringer of Light.

On the one hand, of course, energetic protection against these negative energies is important. On the other hand, learn above all to vibrate higher than what is opposite you. Evil has an important divine mission, if we will.

The psyche as a breeding ground for pattern processing and action initiation is an instance of our brain that becomes relevant much later. It regulates how we deal with certain influences and of course we can help our psyche, which is not exposed to a certain situation for nothing, to align with our own ideas of "good" and "bad". Psychology can help us with this - just like psychologists can. Some people just need it more than others - and that has to do with their karmic pressures, previous actions, and general mental maturity. If you feel that you are evil or subject to constant evil influence, then you need to engage in mental hygiene exercises.

We know that on a spiritual level, we have the eternal law of resonance. So is it "good" to wish a murderer death?

Let's say it depends on how important your own karma is to you and how long you want to experience the supposed duality of good and bad here on earth. Strictly speaking, the earth is probably even a negative form of exception in the universe. A lot of "bad" happens here, but that's why this planet is so special. Here we experience a limitation that is rather atypically high in the universe. If we manage to dissolve them anyway, any species can.

Chapter Four
___

SPIRITUAL ENLIGHTENMENT

Since the dawn of humanity, humans have raised questions and ideas about what spirit is and what it isn't. Some say that the Spirit is God – the beginning of all things. Some say it is the soul – the true self. The truth is, this spirit is your state of consciousness. It is the ability to accept changes (feelings, thoughts, actions, and behavior) in your life.

> *The perfect one is like water*
> *Water provides life for all things*
> *Without competing with anything*
> *Water lives where people hate*
> *Therefore, it can be compared with the Way*
> *Chapter 8 – The Book of Ethics*

A state of consciousness or spirit that follows the Way is flexible (like water). It swells and shrinks. Some events bring joy and goodwill, causing it to swell; others bring pain and sadness, causing it to shrink. The Way is a state of enlightenment first mentioned by Lao Tzu in the Book of Ethics.

Humanity also has a spirit that contracts and expands. When it expands, humanity experiences growth; civilizations flourish, and development occurs. When this collective spirit contracts, the opposite occurs. The most common example of this is the Dark Ages. The church, for whatever reason, felt that its truth, its way, was the only way. However, their way was not the true Way. It was not a state of enlightenment, a state of being and non-being.

> *The highly virtuous people do not pray for virtue;*
> *they already have virtue.*
> *The lowly virtuous people want virtue, so they don't have virtue.*
> *Chapter 38 - The Book of Ethics*

Why Does Spiritual Enlightenment Matter?
When one's spirit reaches a state of flexibility, a state of being and non-being, we say it has attained spiritual enlightenment. But does spiritual enlightenment matter? Why bother with spiritual enlightenment?

An enlightened spirit won't bring about riches because it is neither rich nor poor. It won't make you have plenty because you are neither full nor empty. Instead, the enlightened spirit shows you how to live a happier, longer, and better life.

Searching for happiness
In man's eternal journey, he is always searching for happiness. But the search for happiness is the pursuit of the Way - of spiritual enlightenment. Still, so many people fail to find happiness; why? They look for happiness in the wrong place, and in doing so, they further stray from the Way. You need the discipline to follow the Way.

There is no mystery in finding the Way. All that's required is to keep calm and empty your mind and yourself of every action and desire. When you are empty, you become self-contained. You become valuable to everyone around you. A pot is useful because it is empty. It is what holds our food and lets us cook. We can live in a new house because of the space. If it were full, it would have no value, no use, so like the pot and the new house, we must first empty ourselves. Only then can we find the Way.

As easy as it sounds, finding the Way is almost impossible for most people. The chances of them finding the Way are almost as impractical as seeing pigs fly. Their state of consciousness, their spirit, is yet to expand and attain any form of enlightenment. All they care for is eating and playing.

Life is like a dice game for most people. They place their hopes, dreams, and talents on the dice and hope a roll of the dice will give them all the fortune they desire. That is as far as their spirit has expanded. Their happiness depends on their luck as far as they are concerned.

For some individuals, the Way is something they can almost taste because, on some level, they are aware of this enlightened spiritual state. The problem is they don't know how to achieve it. So they turn to one form of prayer or the other to better tune themselves to the Way. Their true desire is to achieve spiritual enlightenment and embody the way. Yet, it is this desire that keeps them from gaining what they want. Instead of emptying themselves, their thoughts and actions are clouded with desire. They try to reach this enlightened state, so they fill their minds with prayer, but like the pot, they are full, so there's little else they can take in. Until they learn to empty themselves, the Way will remain out of their reach.

The Way is the eternal breath. It is the beginning and the end of all things. If the Way is the beginning and the end, then the Way is in everything, and everything is the Way. The Way is in the sound of nature, the gentlest of breezes, the first light of the morning. To be one with the Way, you need stillness and calm. Stillness, to listen, to hear, and to understand. Prayers and mantras can only take you so far; they often cloud your mind and keep you from the Way.

Close-lipped, breath held
Life is full
Open-lipped, always busy
Life is futile
Chapter 51 – The Book of Ethics

The search for happiness is the search for the Way. Money, fame, wealth, and all worldly desires bring only temporary happiness. True happiness is found in the Way.

An Exercise to Try: learning to listen
The sages of old had to seclude themselves in caves and meditate for years on end before gaining enlightenment and becoming one with the source of all life, the Way. Unless you plan to give up on civilization and become a hermit, that's not possible today. Still, you can try this simple exercise to help you connect with the origin of life.

Find somewhere quiet, sit, or lie down comfortably. Listen to the sounds all around you. Like a rabbit, your mind will wander – let it. The goal is to empty your mind of all thoughts until you are one with the sound surrounding you. Do this for twenty minutes every day for several weeks.

This exercise requires patience. It'll take a while before you can let go of all the thoughts that cross your mind. But pretty soon, you'll find it easy to reach that state, and you will have taken your first steps towards enlightenment.

Chapter Five

THE WAY TO INNER PEACE

Peace is a precious thing
Victory is not something to rejoice about
The one who rejoices in victory is a ferocious man
who likes to kill.
By enjoying killing, one cannot satisfy people.
Chapter 31 – The book of ethics

We have never been more connected than we are today. The internet age is often praised as an age of growth and expansion, yet we have never felt more disconnected as humans. Anxiety, stress, depression, even internet-induced ADD (attention deficit disorder) are issues most of us are familiar with these days.

Most of these issues exist because of an imbalance somewhere in our life, be it a chemical, emotional, or physical imbalance. The most practical solution is therapy for some of these people, but for others, the search for inner peace to quell anxious thoughts and dispel stress.

But is inner peace something you can order from Amazon? Or turn on like a light switch? Inner peace is simply another form of spiritual enlightenment; like all that is part of the Way, attaining inner peace is a lifelong journey that requires your full commitment.

So how do we attain inner peace, and what does inner peace even mean?

Does the Internet leave room for inner peace?

Whether we choose to acknowledge it or not, the internet takes a toll, often a heavy one, on us. The internet never sleeps, and because of that, there's this subconscious pull on most users to stay plugged in for as long as possible. This leads to increasing cases of insomnia, stress, anxiety, and even depression.

The internet can also be rather unforgiving. People are praised for being savage, for dragging others, so much so that it even gave birth to a new form of violence, trolling.

Some might say the internet isn't real; you can just plug it out whenever you feel like it. But the reality is, a huge part of our lives relies on the internet. Our jobs need us to stay connected. We pay our bills on the internet; we get the news on the internet; it feels like there's no room to breathe and slow down. For many people, trying to keep up with the internet traps them in a self-destructive cycle.

One reason for this trap most people have found themselves is that few people are aware of the Way. They are either consuming everything and everything the internet has to offer or giving too much of themselves to the Internet, which leaves no room for the Way.

Does this mean today's society can't find inner peace? No! It simply means it's harder and will require a conscious decision on your part to get it. The search for inner peace must be consistent and active part of your life. You must work for it. It is the only escape out of the chaos of the internet age. As we proceed, you'll learn a few tips that'll help you attain inner peace. You'll also learn how inner peace relates to the Way.

Defining Inner Peace and Its Importance

Whenever people hear the term inner peace, they assume you're referring to something spiritual and relate it to Eastern religions such as Buddhism and Taoism. But inner peace can be practiced by anyone regardless of their religious beliefs.

The reason inner peace is associated with Eastern teachings is that understanding the Way originated in the east. Remember, practicing the Way means embracing inner peace (peace with yourself) and outer peace (peace in your environment). One cannot fully grasp the Way if he/she lacks peace.

Unfortunately, outer peace is something you can't always have control over. As for inner peace, that is completely in your grasp as long as you choose it. Before you can understand inner peace, you have to understand what it isn't.

Inner peace is not:
- Turning down opportunities to try new things, grow your life, or expand your spiritual consciousness.
- Staying passive and watching life pass you by.
- Becoming timid, quiet, meek, or a reserved individual. A lot of people confuse being meek with having inner peace. It is not. The Way is not for the meek.

In other words, inner peace is not about how people see you; just because an individual appears humble does not mean he or she has attained inner peace. Can inner peace influence or change how others perceive you? Absolutely. But first, you need to have reached a state of inner peace. When you reach this state, others will subconsciously recognize that you are becoming one with the Way.

Now that you know what inner peace isn't, it is time to understand what it is. A seeker, one who yearns for the Way, is said to have achieved inner peace when his spiritual and mental bodies are in harmony (more on this later). You may recall that the Way is in all things; the Way is nature, and to hear it and tune into it, you need to calm your mind and empty yourself. Inner peace is this state of calmness. The thoughts in your head slow down and go quiet; the tangled threads in your spirit begin to unravel. Soon you'll be able to sense the state of oneness that is the Way.

The world is a loud place. It's no wonder very few people are even aware of the Way. But when you gain inner peace, the constant noise gradually dims, leaving only silence.

Why does inner peace matter?
Inner peace is important for all sorts of reasons. It is an important foundational step for those seeking the Way. Even if you're not interested in enlightenment, inner peace is still quite useful.

By achieving inner peace, your thoughts grow silent, allowing you to examine yourself fully and discover the problem areas in your life (be it physical or mental)? Those battling stress and anxiety can slowly unravel the thread causing them anxiety or stress. As you cleanse yourself of these burdens, you'll find that your mind is clearer and that your view of life has changed. The journey to inner peace can be a saving grace for millions if only they knew its value. Lucky for you, you've gotten your hands on this book. You've taken the first steps towards becoming a better you.

What does inner peace look like?
I'm sure right now you're asking yourself if inner peace is something internal and not external; how do I know if I've achieved inner peace? You know you've attained inner peace when:

- You don't rely on material things and achievements to be happy and content. Your happiness comes from your connection with your spirit. The stronger the bond, the more content you'll be.
- You've become a complete version of yourself without any new gains.
- You let yourself be whoever you want to be, and you always strive to be the best version of yourself – one that has mental clarity and calm presence that comes with connecting with your spirit.
- You're not bothered, but superficial plans or weighted down by physical worries.
- You accept everything that comes because you know that the Way is everything, so everything that happens is preparing you for the Way.

Six habits Blocking You from Attaining Inner Peace

The road to achieving inner peace is long, the journey is solitary, and some may find the path much easier than others. How you choose to travel on this path varies from one individual to another, not to mention the mental and psychological blocks you need to overcome before you can reach a state of peace as well.

Regardless of how your journey goes, some obstacles are common to anyone looking for inner peace. Most of these obstacles exist because of the age we find ourselves; others exist because the collective spirit of humanity often manifests itself in the same form to everyone (even though most people are ignorant of this global consciousness). Let's take a look at some of these obstacles and how you can overcome them.

1. *Tying your happiness to material gains*

   Thanks to capitalism, people end up measuring their happiness by the number of things they have. This book isn't here to criticize capitalism as far as economies go; it is one of the most successful. However, there's no denying that capitalism has its problems.

   Unfortunately, the happiness that comes from material items is fleeting. Human wants are insatiable, so to tie your happiness to something like that is a recipe for disaster. You may tell yourself I'll be happy when I get this promotion, so you work towards it, and you get it. Soon enough, your lifestyle goes up because of the increase in your income. Before you know it, that moment of joy that came from getting that promotion is gone. This is where anxiety and stress start to come in, and you start waiting for the next promotion before you're happy again.

True happiness comes from within, and yes, that sounds like a cliché, but clichés can be truths. The first step is to connect with your spirit consciously (see the previous exercise); then, you can figure out what you can offer life and get back from life in return.

2. *Running from your emotions*

Growing up, I heard from everyone around me how men don't show emotions because showing emotions made you weak. Sadly, I was an emotional kid, so I ended up burying my emotions because I wanted to be seen by the world as a man, as strong. But, of course, that only caused problems along the way. The emotions I bottled up kept erupting at the worst times.

It wasn't until I discovered the Way that I realized that emotions are a part of us, and to deny them is to deny part of who we are. By denying your emotions, you're creating disharmony within yourself. Society tells us that certain feelings are good and others, such as anger, fear, jealousy, sadness, are inappropriate, and we should hide them. If you truly want inner peace, you have to accept all your emotions, both the "good" and the "bad." Understand why you're feeling those emotions, accept that they're there, but don't let them rule you.

Of all the emotions, the one people struggle with the most is emotion. When people get angry, they deal with it in two ways; suppress it and channel their thoughts positively.

Thinking positive thoughts is an understandable gesture. Many self-proclamation gurus claim the power of positive thinking as the response to anger and other "negative emotions," but why should you have to suppress your anger? The Way is everything, and everything is the Way, which means anger, happiness, sadness, fear, all of that are part of the Way.

Feeling anger on its own isn't a problem. The problem is letting it control you and lashing out because of it. The best way to let go of anger is to understand the source. Once you understand the reason for your anger, you can develop a solution to deal with the problem. The same goes for jealousy, fear, and any other "bad emotion" you might be feeling. The emotion isn't the problem. It's how you deal with it, that is.

Once you've gotten the hang of working your way to the source of your emotions, you'll find that you're one step closer to getting inner peace.

3. *Constantly comparing yourself to others*
   Theodore Roosevelt once said, "comparison is the thief of joy." Comparison is also a major obstacle on the road to inner peace. Modern-day culture is obsessed with comparison. People don't just compare physical items anymore. They compare the number of likes and followers on their social media pages. Some even go as far as crafting fake likes to boost their following and number of likes.

Teenagers fall into depression and become unhappy because their posts on social media are doing fewer numbers than their friends. Unfortunately, there are no exercises that can help you overcome this obstacle quickly. You can only overcome it when you learn contentment.

4. *Placing your self-worth on productivity*
Everywhere you look, you'll see articles, blog posts, and videos on how to increase productivity or how such and such made $10,000 in three days. So it's no surprise that we've gotten the idea stuck in our heads that only when we're productive does our lives have meaning.

The problem is, you can't be productive every minute of the day. You also can't let the achievements of others pressure you and have you believe that your life has no meaning if you're not productive.

Half the time, this idea that we should always be productive stems from being scared of looking like failures to others. So we try to fill up time with activities that end up causing unnecessary stress.

5. *Having low self-esteem*
We can often be our own worst enemies. One major obstacle that hinders us from attaining inner peace is our self-esteem. Self-esteem refers to your sense of self (value). Low self-esteem arises when you lack confidence in yourself and feel bad about yourself. It often causes you to criticize yourself harshly and can even negatively impact your physical and mental wellness.

Low self-esteem will make you feel like you're not good enough and don't deserve the wins in your life. Left unchecked, it can affect our psyche and cause one to start having suicidal thoughts.

No matter who you are or where you're from and regardless of your socioeconomic class, always remember that you matter and you are enough.

6. *Running from our past*

We all have a story to tell, and it's not always a rosy one. It's filled with heartache and pain, regrets, and skeletons in the closet. When you run from your past due to shame or fear, you end up getting chained by memories of your past. You may not feel the effects of these chains, but they are there, constantly affecting your spirit and hindering your growth.

How can you achieve inner peace if you're ashamed of your past? Unless you acknowledge whatever action you did back then and accept that it happened, you're never going to make any progress on this journey to inner peace.

Inner peace means being at peace with all parts of you, including your strengths, weakness, and everything in between. If you try to hide some parts of yourself, it'll be impossible to find inner peace.

The road to Inner Peace

What does the journey to inner peace look like? What does it feel like walking on that road? Is it something you can start and finish in a single day? Is achieving inner peace as simple as flipping a proverbial button?

Inner peace doesn't exist on its own; you can't go to sleep with troubles and wake up the next day content and peaceful. While miracles do happen, they are called miracles for a reason. Ninety nine percent (99%) of the time, you have to work and earn this peace for yourself. Inner peace is not a dial you can just turn anytime you want; it's a process.

Because of the perceived difficulty in achieving inner peace, most people believe you'd have to be spiritual and practice your spirituality for years before attaining inner peace. But inner peace has nothing to do with your level of spirituality.

The reason it's so hard for most people to achieve is they're not willing to accept every part of themselves. There's good in everyone, but there's also much ugly in us too, and for most people, they are unwilling to accept that part of themselves. How can you be at peace if you deny yourself?

We tend to indulge in many self-destructive behaviors that block us from progressing on the road to inner peace. These habits reduce our mental and spiritual energy and redirect our focus on the wrong things, creating disharmony and imbalance within us.

The good news is it takes very little to readjust our energy and daily behavior and put our focus back towards striving for inner peace. Here are some adjustments to change your thinking whenever you feel like the journey is becoming too difficult.

- *Stop blaming yourself*
  To achieve inner peace, you need to accept every action, both good and bad, that you've taken in life. This means taking

accountability and accepting responsibility for your past and present actions. It does not mean blaming yourself for every little thing. You'll only end up appearing self-righteous.

You need to balance accepting responsibility for your actions and recognize that some things are beyond your control.

- *Let go of the victim mentality*
While some excessively blame themselves, others constantly see themselves as a victim. They are always on the lookout for a reason to justify their actions or someone else to blame. These people find it hard to take responsibility for their actions.

Victim mentality causes one to be self-conscious, leading to self-esteem issues, thereby hindering one from finding inner peace. Instead of thinking and acting like it's you against the world, re-examine your actions and take responsibility for situations you caused yourself.

- *Stop people-pleasing*
Another bad habit that you need to let go of if you want an easier time on the road to inner peace is people-pleasing. If you spend your whole life trying to please everyone, you'll end up pleasing no one and lose yourself in the process. Seeking praise and admiration from others prevents you from being your true self and acting with your own will.

Instead of spending all your time and energy trying to gain admiration from others, you're better off learning more about the Way. One with the Way is one with everything. When you know the Way, everything follows.

"By keeping the great Way, the people will follow.
Because the Way is a comfortable and peaceful place
Chapter 35 - *The Book of Ethics*

- *Let go of past grudges*
  Holding on to past grudges is a way of consoling ourselves
  against the hurt we feel. But by holding on, you're only
  stopping yourself from healing and growing. When we're
  mad at people and carry a grudge, in some way, we think
  we're punishing them, but we're only punishing ourselves.

  Why waste your energy on someone who isn't thinking of
  you nor cares about what you think of them? Resentment
  stops you from achieving inner peace because it locks you in
  the past. If you're unable to move on, how will you be able
  to see all the new opportunities and experiences waiting for
  you?

- *Stop trying to be perfect*
  Perfection is another excess that stops you from achieving
  inner peace. When you strive for perfection, you train
  your mind not to settle for anything else, so you're never
  content until you reach whatever level you consider perfect.
  Because of this, they easily give up and only work towards
  things that offer assured self-gratification.

  Some lucky few can use this need to be perfect for motivating
  themselves. They understand that perfection cannot
  be gotten in one go. So they keep on trying, developing
  themselves, working towards perfection. I was not one of
  the lucky ones. My struggle with perfection also created
  self-esteem issues for me. I'd start a project, and no matter

how good it was, I was unhappy because I could not achieve this ideal image of perfection I had in my head. Soon I started feeling like I wasn't good enough; I started attributing my achievements to luck, and I ended up giving up on many things.

It took a while, but after I started on my road to inner peace (and believe me, my journey was not easy), I understood that the idea of perfection I had did not exist. I understood that the only reason I wanted perfection was that I secretly craved the admiration of others. Deep down, I believed I was better than people, and only through creating something perfect could I make everyone see it too. I was small-minded and wanted to feel superior to others. It was only when I stumbled on the teachings of the Way that I could understand all this about myself and take the proper steps to correct this imbalance, find inner peace, and begin my journey to living a better life.

If you also struggle with this, ask yourself why it has to be perfect. Is it for praise? So others will look at you in envy? Why do you chase perfection? If you can't find an answer that isn't toxic, why would you want to spend your life chasing toxicity?

Practical Exercises to attain Inner Peace
Inner peace is like a muscle. It is not a trophy you get and leave on a shelf. Like a muscle, you need to exercise it before seeing any gains and continue exercising to maintain those gains.

Every single person can achieve inner peace. You don't have to be a member of the clergy or a Buddhist monk, or a high-level

Wiccan to achieve inner peace. All that's needed is the will to see the journey to its end. Here are some exercises you may find useful on your journey.

- *Train yourself in the act of mindfulness*
  Being mindful is the process of focusing on a particular thing per time. On the other hand, multitasking is doing several things at the same time. The practice of mindfulness enables you to be fully active, focusing entirely on a single action.

  Besides focusing on a particular thing, mindfulness requires you to be dead to your senses. Being aware of them only leaves you in a constant state of consciousness that is momentary. The Way teaches a state of inner consciousness that is not based on the happenings influenced by external factors. Our inner state controls the outer appearance. As such, being empty in mind with no thoughts preoccupying the inner state is also being mindful. The advantages that are gotten from mindfulness are paramount to our day-to-day activities.

  Mindfulness is the ability to live in the now. It's the ability to be aware of where we are and what we're doing without getting overwhelmed by the external activities going on around us.

  Mindfulness is a great way to learn how to control our actions and emotions, as the state of awareness keeps us from reacting impulsively to whatever is happening.

  You must practice Mindfulness at least twice daily if you want to achieve inner peace. To learn how to practice mindfulness, refer to the nature exercise from earlier. To recap;

→ Find somewhere quiet
→ Pay attention to what's happening in the present
→ Make a mental note of the thoughts that arise, but let them pass by
→ Go back to observing the present
→ Don't judge or criticize yourself regardless of the thoughts that pop up.

When you lose focus and wander while practicing mindfulness, don't let it stress you. When it happens, forgive yourself, put a smile on your face and relax. Check if the wandering brought information or clarity. If it is significant, change your angle, take it that your mind needs a break, readjust your breathing, and continue.

- *Foster Healthy Relationships*
  No one exists in a vacuum, so it's impossible to find inner peace if toxic relationships surround you – and no, I'm not referring to only romantic relationships. Although inner peace happens within, you also need to have a relatively stable and peaceful environment, or you'll find it hard to achieve peacefully.

→ Having healthy relationships around will help you limit the noise and the distractions you're sure to experience daily. So how do you cultivate healthy relationships?

→ Remove toxic people from your life. Anyone that distracts you or directs your thoughts towards unhealthy habits needs to go.

→ Establish healthy boundaries in your personal and professional life, and don't feel bad about holding them.

→ Learn to communicate effectively and let your family and friends know that you're trying to make changes in your life so you'll no longer be able to indulge in certain things.

- *Practice Detachment*
  Detachment teaches you not to take everything so personally. It doesn't mean you don't care; it just means you let go of the idea of trying to force or control a specific outcome. Instead, you surrender yourself to the process and are satisfied with whatever the results are.

  Detachment has nothing to do with being unemotional or distant. It's a state of mind that should be more accurately called "non-attachment."
  "The root of suffering is attachment." - Buddha

By practicing detachment, you'll be able to sit back without fear or worry over a specific outcome because you understand that whatever happens was meant to.

How to Preserve your Inner Peace
Everyday living comes with many distractions and interruptions. One way to shield yourself from all of the chaos of today's society is by practicing inner peace. But achieving inner peace is only one-half of the journey. Recall I said

inner peace is like a muscle, and like any muscle, it'll atrophy if you don't strengthen it every day. How do you strengthen inner peace? Through constant meditation. You also need to safeguard yourself. Otherwise, you may end up falling into old traps and habits.

Watch out for these four mind demons even after you've achieved inner peace.

- *Greed*
  As you get more attuned with inner peace, you will find that the thought bubbles up in your mind to cause a little trouble. This is just greed manifesting itself, and wanting more will only disrupt the level of contentment that you have achieved.

- *Vanity*
  A key concept on the road to inner peace is acceptance. You need to accept who you are, including your failings. It also means accepting criticism when it comes without blaming yourself or trying to play the victim.

- *Fear*
  Achieving inner peace will help you understand the importance of living in the moment. However, you should still be open to whatever the future brings. Fear of the unknown, of uncharted territory, will only cripple all your achievements.

- *Attachment*
  Attachment is what leads to control. You try to control every little detail of your life and the love of others. The only way

to preserve your inner peace is to accept whatever comes and realize that there will always be things you can't predict or control.

Nowadays we are constantly being influenced by different sorts of stimuli, and it is very easy to get distracted by superficial things that really do not give us anything but a waste of time. This is why it is very important to know how to distinguish and identify those things or stimuli that give us energy. They give us something positive or something that we need at the moment. On the other hand, the stimuli that wear us out and take away our energy do not give us anything positive other than wear and tear; energetic, physical and emotional.

Chapter Six

MEDITATION

Today's society has taught us that material things are the only reward in the material world. But as you learned earlier, no material item can give you true peace. Sure, it'll hold your attention for a bit, and for a while, you'll feel like you've achieved something, but eventually, you'll get bored of the item, and it'll lose its appeal. This is how people get stuck in the rat race.

So what's the alternative? Give up on all life? No! You can try meditation instead.

Meditation is about finding peace, love, happiness, and joy within yourself. We all have our inner demons (you can call them inner blocks if you prefer), and these blocks are constantly fighting to tear us apart. With meditation, you can break free from these blocks and the unnecessary wants and desires that keep you trapped in the rat race. In time, meditation will also teach you balance as well as compassion and wisdom. It'll also teach you to let go of your attachments, fear, greed, and whatever mind demon troubles you.

Nobody wants to be a hater, and nobody wants to be in a state of constant anger. Anger is a natural human emotion. Sadly for most people, it makes them miserable and poisons their bodies. Meditation can free you from their clutches. Finding peace today can be harder than finding a needle in a haystack, especially for those without proper guidance.

Meditation helps to connect with your Spirit while clearing out whatever chooses to block this connectivity. One of the primary concerns of the Way is allowing you to connect to the sense of nature and the universe (the Spirit of heaven and earth).

Can you remember the last time you stopped to appreciate the vast sky? We're merely a speck in our universe, yet some people have never thought to look beyond themselves because they've let themselves be trapped by their egos. They're not connected to their innermost self, the Spirit. Since its inception, one of the purposes of meditation has been to connect you with your true self, your Spirit. Some call this connection filled with the Holy Spirit, awakening your soul, or attaining the Buddha state. Whatever you want to call it, it's all about connecting to the inner core with you. The more you meditate, the more your ability to connect your Spirit increases.

The initial goal of the internet was so people could share resources. With time, it grew to become a global connection hub. Yet, people have never been more disconnected from one another. The way you experience life is determined by the lens through which you view it, and for a while, the internet was a new lens that let us view life in different and exciting ways.

But like all material things, it has become shackles on most people. Meditation helps you release whatever inhibits you from experiencing life to the fullest. This doesn't mean you have to disconnect from the internet fully. Like it or not, you're a part of this physical world, so you have to interact with it. Meditation simply lets you take back control. It also gives you a sense of clarity you may have been missing, allowing you to interact with the items of the material world without getting influenced by them.

Many people can't find happiness because they don't feel this connection to their Spirit. They know sometimes it is missing but can't recognize what it is. Connecting with your Spirit, finding the Way, can turn a fool into a wise man. Meditation allows you to relax at the center of your being, allowing you to find balance and learn compassion for others.

Fusing Your Life Experiences to Become a Better You
How many notifications did your phone get today? Add to that the number of random information you come across, and you'll agree with me that we often experience an information overload daily. What happens when you overload a computer? First, the processing speed slows down; it warns you to close some applications, and if the overload remains, it starts overheating and may eventually shut down. The same thing happens to us. The only difference is you do not hear the warning signs because there's so much noise in our consciousness that we can't tell what's important and what isn't.

Humans are complex creatures. Our experiences are horrible and wonderful. For every joyful experience, there's a stressful one. To center ourselves, we need to fuse these experiences. In order words, you need to accept both the horrible and the wonderful if you want peace, and this is where meditation comes in. Not only does it help you sort out all the noise and clean up our system, but it also helps in allowing us to accept every part of ourselves.

We may live in a more civilized society today, but the people of old were more in tune with the Way, the natural breath of life. Today, society is constantly in a rush that people don't even know this breath exists. This constant rush means your mind and body are always active. When your mind can't rest, it goes wild, and when your body can't rest, it gets agitated, further stressing the mind. Before you know it, you're stuck in a negative feedback loop, and your body reacts with a full-blown stress response. When this happens, you may find yourself losing sleep.

Eventually, your emotional state crumbles, and you start having emotional outbursts with no warning. The people around you start asking how this happened, and the sole reason for that is because your bodies – mental and physical – are out of balance. You failed to let all the noise coming from the outside digest, which in turn caused your mental body to be overstimulated. To digest all of this new information and new experiences, you need to meditate.

What Is Meditation?

People say they're meditating, especially new-age yogis, but as wonderful as it sounds, hearing it doesn't exactly describe what they're supposed to be doing. It's like when people say they

INSIGHTS TO BETTER LIVING

pray. You don't ask if they're praying to God, an angel, the Devil, or the owner of their favorite restaurant. You just smile, nod, and say, "Oh, that's wonderful that you pray." Just hearing that they meditate or pray is enough.

Many forms of meditation do indeed exist, but Westerners mix up meditation with contemplation. They think meditation is when you place all your thoughts on something. So if you think about an idea, westerners say, you're meditating on the idea. But from an Eastern point of view, thinking about an idea isn't meditation; that's an analysis.

True meditation looks more like philosophy to those in the western world. But even then, while they appear similar on the surface, they're completely different. Philosophy is defined as the study of the basic ideas about knowledge, right and wrong, reasoning, and the value of things. Eastern philosophy looks at ideas like reincarnation and karma, while western philosophies examine ideas about good and evil, specifically God, heaven, and hell. Meditation isn't concerned with examining ideas. It is a process of connecting with your Spirit and releasing the blocks accumulated in your mind and body.

The reason most people fail at meditation is that they come at it with the wrong mindset. They start meditating because they expect to get something from mediation when meditation is the ability to let go. As long as you start meditating only so you can obtain something, you'll never get anything out of it. Expectations have no place in meditation. Buddha never meditated to get something. He did it to get free of the need for things, and that's the key. Meditation isn't to help you get things. It's to free you from those desires.

As we proceed, we'll look at the Water method of Taoist meditation as described in the book of ethics – the teachings of the Way. Spiritual enlightenment starts with improving your body, hence the first part of this book. Once you become fully relaxed and your physical health is in peak condition, you can then start working to connect with your Spirit.

Making Sure Your Expectations are Balanced

One who acts fails
One who holds loses
Therefore:
Sage doesn't act
Thereupon he doesn't fail
Doesn't keep
Thereupon he doesn't lose
Chapter 64 – The Book of Ethics

Another aspect of meditation that is crucial for spiritual enlightenment is that it relieves you of the weight of expectations. We've been conditioned from a young age to keep up with external expectations constantly. It gets to a point, and you can't even remember why those expectations matter at all. Expectations don't lead to inner peace or longer, better life.

Expectations are rooted in power, and like everything else in life, they have their pros and cons. The physical world is filled with all kinds of scientific marvels and inventions, and your expectations help you take advantage of them. However, having expectations in your inner world can create conflict within yourself. Meditation helps you manage your expectations. The meditation method that we will learn will help you let go of expectations. You can move from where you are to where you want to be by casting off those burdens. With enough practice, you may eventually arrive at the goal of Spiritual Enlightenment or, as the Christians would say, directly commune with God.

The Water Method of Meditation
Under the dome of the sky, nothing is softer than water.
But the hard-hitting attack is nothing more
So nothing can replace it
Chapter 78 – The Book of Ethics

One of the main tenets of the Way is fostering spontaneity. Most people have lost the spirit of spontaneity because so many expectations tie them down. People care more for how they look on the outside yet spend little time taking care of their inner selves. The Way considers humans as being one with nature, even though they're unaware of it, so the first step in learning the way is connecting with your true self, and this is where meditation comes in. The Way does not believe or promote any God. If anything, it celebrates all God as one with nature. The only concern is freeing people from their internal struggle and helping them reach spiritual enlightenment.

Inner versus Outer Wealth
There are more churches, alternate religions, and spiritual practices than they were a decade ago. Thousands of years ago, religion wasn't as mainstream as it is now. People were free to practice in whatever and whoever they wanted. Yet, with so many religions around, people today seem to be far from spiritual enlightenment and inner peace than people of old.

Sadly, most religions today prioritize the gospel of prosperity over one of spiritual enlightenment. They preach the story of wealth and say that by joining them, you'll unlock your riches, get powerful, basically feeding into your desires. They address the issue of external riches. Meditation is concerned mainly with enriching the inner and using that to make your outer life better.

We live in a physical world, so of course, external wealth is important. You need money to get access to food, clothing, shelter, a good education, and a host of other things. But developing your inner self, your Spirit, is more important than chasing external wealth.

It is the strength of your Spirit that will allow you to ride the ups and downs that litter the road of life. So how do you cultivate inner wealth? Through the meditation of course. In time you'll find that you're happier, not because you're richer or because of any change in your external circumstance, but because you can finally sense the connection with nature that you've been missing all this time. You can use the water method of meditation to find clarity, connect with nature, and attain spiritual enlightenment.

What is the Water Method of Meditation?
Ancient Chinese had a philosophy that described the nature of all things. They called this philosophy the yin-yang philosophy. The philosophy states that the universe has a dualistic nature composed of two complementary and competing forces, dark and light, male and female, hot and cold, hard and soft. The ancient Chinese also created meditation techniques based on

this philosophy, namely the fire meditation method and the water meditation method. The fire method of meditation corresponds with the Yang force; it is a hard technique where one changes and attempts to connect to their inner self through hypnosis.

The water method is based on the Yin philosophy and is a soft method of meditation. It teaches release, that is, releasing everything harmful and unnecessary from your life. It preaches letting go.

Lao Tzu first introduced the water method of meditation in his Book of Ethics and, since then, has gained popularity both in China and across the globe thanks to the growth of Taoism (the practice born from the book of ethics). Part of why the water style of meditation is so popular maybe because we yearn to be like water, soft yet powerful deep down. Water is so powerful that mere sound, sight, and even touch are enough to bring most people into a peaceful state.

Water as a style of meditation may be so appealing because deep down, we yearn to be more like it. Its effects are so powerful that the mere sight, sound, or touch of it alone is enough to bring us into a peaceful state.

Another reason it's so popular is that we're water bodies. The average human is 60% water; even the earth we live on is made up of water (about 70%). There's no doubt that we're connected to this life-giving liquid on a fundamental level.

Water also plays an important role in various religions and cultures. It signifies purity, clarity, and calmness.

The Christians use water when carrying out baptism to symbolize purification and being reborn through Christ. In Islam, water is seen as sustaining and life-giving. Giving water to another living is seen as a noble and greatly rewarded act. The Japanese Shinto religion uses water in its purification rituals. They view water as a symbol for the flow of life. The Hindus also view water as a means of purifying and washing away sins.

In Taoism, the Chinese tradition founded by Lao Tzu, the writer of the book of ethics, water represents dissolution. That is dissolving blocks, negative emotions, and connecting with nature.

How Does Water Meditation Work?
Water provides life for all things
Without competing with anything
Water lives where people hate
Therefore, it can be compared with the Way
Chapter 8 – The Book of Ethics

The water method of meditation works by stilling the mind and focusing on the inner. It is a yin-based meditation method that uses awareness to dissolve or wash away all the blocks and negative energies that have accumulated in our bodies. This form of meditation allows you to awaken your Spirit (sometimes called soul, life-energy, or chi). By practicing this water meditation regularly, you'll be able to:

- Calm the mind
- Harmonize your body, mind, and spirit (more on harmonies later)

- Release physical and mental traumas
- Free yourself from anxiety and stress.
- Relax your nervous system
- Be more open-minded to all that life has to offer
- Become more productive
- Live a longer life
- Become more adaptable

Benefits of Water Meditation?
Water meditation is a straightforward practice if you know what you're doing. Most of the benefits have already been stated earlier. However, to emphasize the importance of water meditation, here are some more benefits.

- It helps to improve concentration and focus.
- It helps in improving your mental state.
- It'll leave you feeling healthier and full of energy.

Exercise to Try - 3 Breathing Techniques
One way to develop an awareness of the energies inside you is through internal breathing. You can practice this technique while standing or sitting. Remember to always breathe through your nose unless you need to breathe through your mouth due to some medical condition.

There are three breathing techniques for you to try. They can benefit you in so many ways. Before you get started, you should remember to:

→ Stay relaxed, especially in your face, neck, jaw, and shoulder areas.
→ Use the tip of your tongue to gently touch the roof of your mouth while practicing any of these breathing exercises.

→ Go with an attitude of curiosity and patience. Try to stay focused on the practice without creating any tension.

- *Abdominal Breathing*
  The first breathing technique is known as abdominal breathing. Start by finding somewhere comfortable to sit, preferably in an upright position. Close your eyes and pay attention to the movement of your breath. Observe your inhalations and exhalations without trying to alter their natural rhythm. Follow this breath for ten cycles.

  Next, form a triangle with your fingers over your navel. Taoists call this area the lower tan tien (or dantian). To form the triangle, gently place your hands on your lower abdomen. Let the tips of your thumbs touch each other directly over your navel while your first fingers do the same a few inches below.

  To practice the abdominal breathing technique, let the lower portion of your abdomen, the part beneath your fingers, gently expand with each inhale, and relax back to its natural position when you exhale. That's all there is to it. You inhale, expand, then exhale, and relax. Repeat this process for ten cycles.

- *Reverse Breathing*
  As always, sit upright in a comfortable position, then follow along with the natural rhythm of your breath. Repeat this for ten cycles without trying to change its rhythm or quality in any way.

  Form a triangle with your hands (see abdominal breathing technique) and place it over your lower abdomen. As you inhale, let your lower abdomen, the part beneath your fingers, contract inward towards your spine. Reverse breathing is the opposite of abdominal breathing, hence the name. As you contract your abdomen, you may feel a gentle inward and upward scooping sensation. Take note of this sensation. As you exhale, allow your abdomen to expand outward to its natural position.

Once again, you contract your abdomen on the inhale and expand on the exhale. Repeat this for ten cycles of breath.

- *Vase Breathing*
  Vase breathing is a variant of abdominal breathing with some reverse breathing added to the mix, and to top it off, a visualization technique. The vase starts the same as the other two by following the natural rhythm of your breath for ten cycles and placing your hands over your lower belly in a triangle shape.

  As you inhale, allow your lower abdomen to expand outwards and touch your hands (see abdominal breathing). While inhaling, picture your torso as a vase, and every time you inhale, the vase is being filled with fresh, clean water. The water fills the base (your lower abdomen) first and then gets to the brim (your collarbone).

  Allow your abdomen to relax back to its natural state as you exhale. Since vase breathing is more complex than the other two, your best bet is to get familiar with those two first. Also, instead of doing ten cycles, you can do two, three, or four cycles till you're comfortable and familiar with the practice.

How to Calm the Monkey Mind

Most people that are trying meditation for the first time usually have the same complaint. Their minds keep wandering, and they can't stay focused. This is a common problem today. We live in a fast-food society, meaning we want everything immediately. Our mind gets addicted to this instant gratification that comes with living in such a society.

Your mind can get you in plenty of trouble if you start using it to think instead of just observing; in other words, you've allowed the monkey mind to lead. The monkey mind gets us into trouble because it always seeks stimulation, jumping from one thought or idea to another. As a result, we get involved in things we're not supposed to because of the monkey mind and our egos.

But the mind isn't the villain here, and we certainly can't destroy it. It's a part of us. So what do we do with it? How do we get the monkey mind to sit still? There are many ways to handle the monkey mind. We'll be looking at one of the ways you can get the monkey mind to go where you want and do what you want. The monkey mind loves stimulation, so that's what we're going to use. We'll give the mind what it loves; an activity to focus on. Soon it'll get lost in the activity, and before you know it, the monkey mind will finally quiet.

Instead of trying to empty your mind, which is almost impossible, the trick is to let the mind participate in the mediation. This won't be easy; we're already conditioned to letting the mind get its way. But little drops make an ocean, and practice makes perfect. At first, the mind will resist and try to jump elsewhere, but in time it'll come to accept meditation as one of its favorite activities. By getting the monkey mind to do many things at once, it'll end up losing itself. You'll find the yin (the emptiness, the connection to the way) through the yang (activity). This is how to calm the mind. You slow it down with various activities to connect to the energy inside, the emptiness, and nature.

Once you learn to lead the monkey mind, you'll stop thinking with your mind and start thinking with your inner self, the heart. Letting the monkey mind lead is like driving a car a hundred miles per hour. If you were to look outside, all you'll see is a blurry landscape. But if you stop the car and walk, you'll be able to take in everything. This is what meditation teaches, and it's what you get when you calm your monkey mind. You'll be able to see the big picture, observe all that's happening around you instead of letting the monkey run around. When the monkey leads, you end up living a reactionary life, and you'll never really accomplish all that you want in life.

What makes the monkey mind so interesting is that it loves playing tricks, which is how it traps you all the time. But if you know how, then you can turn the tables on the mind. Instead of chasing the monkey, you let it come to you. There's a saying, "to catch a monkey, stick a banana in a jar, and the monkey will come for the banana." The monkey mind functions in the same vein; it'll stick its hand in the jar and reach for the banana. So now the monkey has a banana in its hand but can't get said hand out of the jar. It can easily take its hand out if it lets go of the banana, but the mind won't, and that's how you end up trapping the monkey mind.

The monkey mind is associated with the ego, and the same way you trap the monkey with the banana is the same way we get trapped when the monkey, the ego, leads. The monkey mind will rather hold on to the banana than let go even for its freedom. As you're reading this, I'm sure you can recall situations that could have been solved easily if only you had let go, but you refused because of your ego. Now you know why that is; you were letting the monkey lead.

This is how you get the monkey mind to relinquish control. You get it focused on an activity, and it'll forget where it is, what it was doing, and finally, it'll forget why it was leading. And just like that, you have tricked the monkey mind into becoming dormant.

This is exactly what the ancient Chinese sages did when they practiced meditation. They give the monkey mind what it loves most – activity. Then they trap the mind in one area with the activity. Soon enough, by giving the mind all that activity, it'll forget itself.

The sages used to keep the monkey mind busy by getting it to try and trace the thirty-two energy channels in the body. You can try something different and have the monkey mind focus on the rhythm of your breathing, or you could picture a ball of light at the location of your third eye (also known as the inner eye or mind's eye) and have the monkey swim towards it. You'll soon see that the monkey mind easily gets lost in its activity. That is how you get the monkey mind to participate in your meditations actively.

Calming the monkey mind is good for more than just meditation practice. You'll find that you can focus more on your regular life. You can think clearer, but more importantly, you'll realize that you're one step closer to the Way. As the monkey mind starts to lose itself, it'll enter into the void (the Way). When that happens, you'll be able to observe the nothingness of nature and communicate with your Spirit. So next time the monkey starts jumping all over the place, just smile and direct it where you want it to go and watch as it leads you into the Way.

The Way of Tao

> *The Way is empty but not used up*
> *The deep Way is like the root of all species.*
> *The Way blunts the sharp*
> *The Way unties the trouble*
> *The Way softens the glare*
> *The Way harmonizes with the dust*
> *The Way is dark, but it seems to exist*
> *I do not know who the children of the Way are.*
> *But the Way appeared out before heaven and earth*
> *Chapter 4 – The Book of Ethics*

Becoming one with the Way requires our mental, emotional, and physical bodies to be in harmony. This harmonization occurs through three stages; concept, desire, and manifestation. The Way is simple, think, and it happens. But how do you harmonize your bodies? What do concept, desire, and manifestation mean?

We are made up of three bodies: the physical body (the one everyone is aware of), the mental body, and the emotional body. These bodies follow a sort of structural hierarchy. The mental body manages the emotional body, while the emotional body controls the physical body. So when we talk of concept, desire, and manifestation, we mean using our mental (to create a concept), emotional (to desire that concept), and physical (manifesting the desires) in tandem.

Here's how it works. Any action you take starts with an idea or a concept, and the concept (the mental body) controls the emotional body. The emotional body is the desire to make it happen, while the physical manifests that desire.

Although you may not be familiar with the idea of three bodies, the idea isn't new. Mainstream media marketers and self-proclaimed gurus call it the power of positive thinking. What is positive thinking of not creating a concept and generating a positive thought to produce the desired result? The difference is most people didn't know how it worked, which is why they found it hard to apply it in the first place.

Like Napoleon Hill once said, "What the mind can conceive and believe, the mind can believe."

When your mental body gets the concept, you'll gain understanding, and from there, your emotional body creates desire, giving you results. Without this process, you'll not be able to accomplish anything. This manifestation can take a while, and it can happen almost instantly. It all depends on how good you are at conceptualizing your mental body and activating the emotional body to get what you want. The more your practice, the better you'll get, and you'll be able to get your results faster.

This is how you practice the Way. Because the Way is nothing and everything, you'll find that most people already do this, only, they are unaware of what they're doing.

Human creations and technology all start as a concept, then a blueprint is created, and that blueprint goes into engineering and manufacturing. Finally, the components are assembled in a factory. We do the same thing in our daily lives but without the awareness of what we're doing.

When you become conscious of the Way, you'll find that manifesting becomes quicker. All manifesting is, is connecting to the Way. One with the Way has everything and nothing. So the more you practice, the stronger your connection becomes and the better you'll be at manifesting.

The Value of Nothingness

The softest thing in the universe
Wins the hardest in the universe
Emptiness can get into space because there is a gap
So one knows the value of nothingness
Chapter 43 – The Book of Ethics

What is nothingness? Nothingness is the Way, and the Way is everything. So nothingness is everything. When you stand in the middle of nothing, you're actually in the presence of all things. Everything comes from nothingness.

"In the beginning was the Word, and the Word was with God, and the Word was God." - John 1:1

The Bible verse above tells us that everything came from nothing. In this case, nothingness is considered the word, and the word was God, and God created the world. You can also see it in science with the big bang theory, the explosion that birthed all life. To go into nothingness is to return to this nothingness (because we all started from nothingness). This nothingness is God, the Way, infinity. Words are not enough to explain it.

The Way – cannot be told.
The Name – cannot be named.
The nameless is the Way of Heaven and Earth.
Chapter 1 – The Book of Ethics

Trying to use words to explain this nothingness (sometimes known as the infinity God) creates limitations, so you see why nothingness is beyond all words. Lao Tzu called it the Way because he knew the monkey mind would obsess over calling "it" a name, so he called it the Tao (meaning Way).

The Taoist version of creation sounds similar to the big bang theory. A concept thrown into the empty space of the universe was reflected out, hence the bang. A collective thought (or energy) was formed, and this thought was sent into the nothingness, the universe, and it was reflected like light reflecting from a mirror. Creation, and the big bang, is the first known manifestation process. This is how we can manifest everything from nothing because we came from nothing in the first place.

Once you can understand and master this, fully connect with the Way, you'll be amazed by what you can accomplish. All of life is connected; all of life is one. When we form a thought and send it into the universe, we're simply borrowing energy from the collective to manifest it in the physical. You can practice this for a few minutes each day, and with time, it'll manifest in the physical plane. It'll appear when you least expect it. Whatever we want, you can manifest it, whatever the thought, concept, or configuration.

The original act that led to the creation of the universe is something we put into practice, at least subconsciously, through thought every day. But with a clearer understanding of what we're doing and why we are doing it, our focus increases, allowing us to send stronger thoughts into the universe, which it sends back and manifests here in the physical plane. The more we practice, the faster we'll be at manifesting our desires. When we practice every day, we are honing our awareness, making us more conscious of this manifestation. Without practice, we are blind to what we manifest. It never looks like what we want because our monkey mind has confused us with too many distractions, and we lose sight of what we wanted in the first place.

You must be careful with your thoughts, especially when you are conscious of this ability. Whatever thought you send out to the universe will be reflected in you. Ignorance will no longer be an excuse as you are aware of your ability to manifest anything. As you think, so you will become.

When people pray to God (in whatever form they believe in), they're sending their energy out to the heavens and expecting an answer to their prayers. Sometimes their prayers are answered, but for different reasons than what they think. Prayer is asking God for something, a solution to your problems, money, a new car, a new job, a house, whatever it is. In reality, when people pray, they're sending out their energy. Some prayers are answered because the person sending them has a strong desire to reflect the energy and manifest it here. If you understand how and why prayers work and focus properly, praying will be more effective for you.

If nothing is everything, and God is everything, then we are God. The ability to manifest is something we all have within ourselves, and we just don't know it because we forget who we are. Some people don't think prayers work; others think it's ineffective or depends on something arbitrary, like luck when they don't understand the concept. It's not enough to just send a thought out to the universe. You have to put your energy into it. It is this energy that the Christians call faith. Without this energy, nothing will happen.

The same thing happens everywhere, even with black magic practices. People fear witches and wizards because they believe these witches or wizards have power over them when they're the ones feeding it their energy. They strongly believe that a witch/wizard has power over them, so they send that energy out to the universe, and so what happens? It reflects back, and that belief is manifested as black magic. All prayer, all manifestation happen because of you. You are the creator and the one manifesting, it's all our energy. When you send your energy out, the universe multiplies it and reflects it to you, but it's still your energy, just supercharged so it can manifest your desire in the physical.

Chapter Seven

SELF-REALIZATION: DISCOVERING WHO YOU ARE

Self-realization is the process of fully connecting with the Spirit. It is rediscovering what we already know but are not conscious of. The road to self-realization is a slow one due to the fact the road leads nowhere. There's no destination because what you need to discover lies within. It is the journey into nothingness, into infinity. Infinity is never ending but a continuum. For the unaware, it means continuously becoming. It's like climbing a mountain, and your motivation is getting to the top. But on getting there, you realize there's another peak, and on and on, you continue climbing, reaching for peak after peak. This is the nature of infinity - having no beginning and no end.

Those who have discovered their true selves and reached the goal of self-realization are aware of one truth; if infinity has no beginning and no end, then there's no point in that never-ending climb. Wherever you are is where you need to be.

The rat race is another name for this continuum. People get trapped in this rat race because they're always trying to get to the next peak and the one after that. They say to themselves, "Oh, I just need this car, and I'll be happy, or I just need to finish this project, and I'll spend more time with my family." The monkey mind keeps creating peaks for them to reach, and they fail to realize they're stuck in a continuum.

Another truth the mind tries to keep from you is that whatever you want from life will always chase you, especially if you understand how to manifest. But you get so busy running the rat race that your wants and desires can never catch up to you. If you stop running for a moment and take some time to discover yourself, find inner peace, or even do some meditation exercises, you'll find that things you want from life come to you.

The highly virtuous people do nothing
Yet nothing is undone
The lowly virtuous people always do
Yet many more things need to be done
Chapter 38 - The Book of Ethics

This is the secret to living in the Way. It is an effortless way of living. As you become more comfortable with meditation, you'll get one step closer to self-realization. As you learn to tame the mind, you'll slowly start to recall all you have forgotten about the Self. This process of self-realization can only happen when you meditate and find inner peace.

There's a popular saying in the West, "No pain, no gain." It means you can only achieve something through hardships(pain). But the Way teaches us that if there is pain, then there's something wrong. Pain is the body's alarm system. It tells us that we're going against the flow - the natural order of things. We learn to go with the flow on the road to nothing to achieve equilibrium with nature. The Way teaches you to swim on your own, it shows you the path, but you must walk on it yourself. The journey into nothingness is one of self-discovery, so how can anyone teach you? You know yourself best; you know what is inside you, what you're feeling, and what you're going through. No instructor will have that knowledge, so you can only get direction from your lessons.

Teaching yourself also has its benefits. You become more self-sufficient and energetically independent in all aspects of your life. You'll have clarity in all you do because you know what you're going through and can tell what you need to solve it. As you progress in your journey of self-realization, your connection with your mental and emotional bodies also improves, and so does your ability to manifest.

According to Taoist religion, there are three paths to enlightenment. The first is through prayer and worship, the second is through good deeds, and the third is the Way. The first and second can help people reach enlightenment, but you won't know why it'll happen, when it'll happen or how it'll happen. The third path is self-discovery, and you know the why, the when, and the how.

We have mentioned the monkey mind several times in the last chapter and this one. The monkey mind is your greatest obstacle on the path of self-realization. You are part and parcel of the divine, of infinity, but you don't remember who you are. The monkey mind (your ego) draws you away from your true self and traps you in its system of thinking. It draws you away from the path of self-realization and interrupts your connection with the Way. But the monkey mind is not an enemy; it is a part of you. On the path of self-realization, you first have to acknowledge the monkey mind and learn to work with it.

Once you understand how the monkey mind works and realize that it is only your ego, you can take power from it. Remember, nothing happens if you don't give it power. The reason the monkey mind can run amok is that we empower it. The moment you take back that power, you'll be able to direct it to work for you and not against you.

Becoming Your Own Teacher
The beauty of the Way is that it helps you understand that enlightenment is in your hands. Spiritual independence is encouraged as you progress and get closer to nothingness (the Way). You are your own teachers. The exercises and formulas are only there to guide you. You are the only person that can understand what you're going through. Your friends cannot, your parents can't, and no Guru on the internet promising you enlightenment for a monthly subscription can understand. The journey into nothingness is an individual one, and only you can lead yourself to self-realization.

Every individual is unique. You had a one-in-six-trillion chance at life, and you won. There is no one else in this world with the same combination as you. The journey into nothingness also teaches us that there are no enemies or friends in life, only teachers. They are in our lives to teach us what we need to learn, just as we are in their lives to do the same. Everybody around you and every situation you go through teaches you something new about yourself.

There are many roads in life. The Way teaches us that the path to enlightenment means following the middle path. But we must pay attention to what's happening on the left and the right, or we will end up getting lost. If you don't know where the left and right are, how will you know you're walking the middle path? The left and right paths are the two extremes of life, our greatest teachers, calling them friends or enemies, fail to describe their role in our journey to nothingness accurately. The extremes teach us what we need to know about ourselves because they only reflect what we need to learn. This is why we're our own teachers. Everything we need to learn is already around us, and all that's needed is the awareness and the discipline to take the first step. The thing with religion is you're giving your energy to someone else, meaning you lose some of your energy. Although you may learn some new information, you don't learn anything new about yourself. When you give out your energy, you're putting your growth in someone else hands, and it is up to them to use your energy to take care of you or not. You don't lose the energy, but you're giving away your freedom and responsibility to someone else.

If you learn to take care of yourself, then there's one less person to take care of, and that's how you help everyone else. As you learn to take care of yourself and learn how to take responsibility for yourself, there will be no reason to give your energy to anyone else. If someone comes to you in an earnest, respectful, and sincere way, seeking the truth from you, then it's perfectly okay to share the concepts and ideas. When you give out your energy to a master, guru, or religious teacher, you're leaving your spiritual growth in the judgment and mercy of others. Their limited understanding will be what determines your fate. This is not a position to be in, it makes you codependent and leaves you relying on others for discoveries and understanding you can get yourself. The worst part is they can never truly figure out what's best for you because they can't see inside you to know what you need. The only one who knows what's best for you is you.

The Little Pine Trees
The sages of old likened our progress on the Journey into nothingness to the growth of a little pine tree. At first, it seems like the pine trees aren't growing, but if you give it time, you'll find that they are fully grown - bigger and taller than a two-story house. Because you kept looking at the pine trees, it felt like they weren't growing. But after some time, you could see the whole transformation and appreciate the time it took to get there. This is what happens in the journey into nothingness. By practicing the meditation and manifestation techniques slowly over time, the transformation will happen. This change is often so subtle that you don't even realize it's happening until one day, you take a look, and there are two big pine trees inside you.

When you keep up with the practices, your life will change even without you noticing as you connect with your Spirit and achieve self-realization. Since it happens so subtly, you won't even realize the changes are occurring. If you plant a tree and every other minute you're digging it up to check up on it, it'll never grow. It's the same thing that happens on your journey. If you are constantly looking for changes, you are "uprooting" all your progress. Next thing you know, you're wondering why it isn't working. This obsession with monitoring your growth comes from the monkey mind doing what it does best, causing mischief.

The pine tree didn't do anything special to grow as big as it did. It simply went with the natural order of things, absorbing water from the rain, sunshine and going with the universe's flow. This is what the Way tries to instill in us. To connect with your inner self is to go with the flow of the universe. If you do only that, you'll see that anything else you may ever want will follow you.

In the first chapter, we practiced an exercise to help us listen to nature because the answer to all your questions about the Way can be found in nature. A forest can reveal the natural flow of the universe. As you look at the tree, a seed drops down, burrows itself into the ground, and disappears. At first, it seems like nothing is happening, but the seed is flowing into the universe. It is rooting itself in the soil and then after six months it breaks the surface of the soil and becomes a little pine tree. In six months to a year, it becomes a pretty-good-sized tree. It becomes a big tree in ten to fifteen years; then after thirty, forty, fifty years, it is a huge tree; and in seventy to eighty years, it is a gigantic tree. A hundred years later, that little seed becomes a big pine tree that everyone can see from miles away. No one sees the hundred years that led to its growth; all they see is a big pine tree.

Spiritual enlightenment is similar. You may not show any outer progress, but there's a little seed growing. Like every seed, it needs nurturing, and this particular seed gets its nurturing from the practice we do each day. A little bit of water, some sunshine, and before you know it, our seed of enlightenment turns into a big pine tree.

What happens if you expose a seed to too much sun and give it too much water? It dies. Moderation is key, so we say that progress on this journey to self-realization, to nothingness, only requires a little bit of practice. Five to ten minutes of practice every day is enough to turn the seed inside you into a big pine tree.

Chapter Eight
_____

THE WAY OF HAPPINESS

What is happiness?
It is to be satisfied with what you have, accept things without trying to force them and change the consequences, and find beauty in anything.

It's a state you can reach right now, without having to move, do or say anything. It comes from understanding the Way and knowing oneself.

Happiness is an inner state that is easy and simple and requires just a little change in your mindset and the way you look at things.

Happiness is right here, at this very moment. It's in you and everywhere around you. It's in the things you love doing, in the things you have but take for granted, in being kind to others and sharing what you have. From this, we can say that happiness is contained in the Way.

The Road to Happiness

If someone walked up to you right now and asked, "Are you happy?" Will you be able to say yes? Happiness, like everything else, is a personal journey. No one can tell you if you're happy or not, it's something you know for yourself. Happiness, like inner peace, is not something you can win in a lottery. It's not something you stumble into. It is a conscious decision that you have to make constantly.

If you're not happy with someone, then there is no point in keeping that relationship. If you're not happy with your job, quit. If you're happy with the body, you have and don't want to do anything to change it, okay then. It's all about whether it makes you happy or not. That's the ultimate technique when in doubt or have to make an important decision.

The problem is that most of us don't know how to be happy. We may try to find happiness, fix our current situation, or change things. But eventually, we find ourselves in the same old state - wondering if we're happy. This happens because they are stuck in the continuum, so they keep repeating the same mistakes over again.

Here are the three mistakes and how to overcome them:

- *Trying too hard*
  People think they need to do something to be happy, so they start working too hard, pushing themselves to the limit, expecting too much, waiting for happiness to come, and so on. While most people can't recognize this trap for what it is, those of us practicing the Way can tell it is just another trap by the monkey mind to lure you into the continuum.

At some point, you begin to realize you've spent a lifetime trying to reach a certain state when it was in front of your eyes the whole time. What's most beautiful about being happy is that you feel perfect because you're okay with everything, it's like being in sync with everything. Most importantly, you're grateful. You find that things have become easy and they are just the way they should be, so you don't need to make any extra effort, put too much pressure on what you do, or make it harder and more complex than it should be. Look around you and really reflect on how you've gotten to this point. Let go of the pressure you've brought into your life, and things might just get better.

- *It's a place*
  What many people think is that happiness is a goal, a destination, or something out there, or they will reach it in the future. They think it's a goal to be accomplished and they will feel great when it's done, and everything will be fine. This is wrong and never happens, because the future never actually comes. What's even worse is that if you had some kind of a deadline, when you reach it, you would be grossly disappointed because things just wouldn't be the way you expected. You will then begin aiming at something else, trying to find a satisfaction that will never come.

You cannot find happiness anywhere else but right now. Happiness is now. It is right here, and nothing will be different even after a decade if we remain blind to what you presently have. Happiness is not dependent on what goals you accomplish, so when you connect it with something you are looking forward to in the future, you are denying that it's now.

You need to stop making so many goals and plans, spend less time in the future, and live more in this present moment, because happiness is right here and right now, and it's your up to you to decide if you'll enjoy it or let it go.

- *It is in material items*
  Some people try to raise their level of happiness by either buying stuff, going to different places, hanging out, having one relationship after another in the bid to find the perfect one. Or worse - by overeating, drinking alcohol excessively, using drugs, getting immersed online etc.

It may work for a while, but later you'll realize you've created a much larger void inside of you. Now the only way to fill that void is to keep indulging in those excesses. This is a self-destructive behavior, and you will never feel better for real unless you realize you need to make some changes from the inside out.

Happiness is an inner state. It doesn't matter what we have, what we do, who we meet, and how we fill our time. The only crucial thing that defines our happiness (or the lack of it) is how we react to things and our attitude towards life. Do we actively enjoy our lives, are we in harmony with ourselves, and are we full of appreciation for all of life?

Finding Happiness

If the Way is happiness, does that mean anyone not following the Way will never be happy? Of course not. You can still find yourself even if you don't devote yourself to the Way. The difference is in your state of awareness. By reading the rest of this chapter, you can still find happiness (whether or not you're a seeker of the Way).

The 4 Step Plan to Finding Happiness

Many people often ask, "how do I become happy?" Such a simple question with an even simpler answer: *just be.* Be one with nature, with the universe, with life.

That's all it takes to be happy. That is how it works. And yet, we know so many people that have everything they want, everything it takes to be happy no matter what your definition of happiness and success is, but still don't feel satisfied, don't feel like they have a reason to be grateful for, take everything for granted and just aren't happy.

Some people have less than the average person, but it's more than enough for them. And they are way happier than those who have more. It's simply because they appreciate it and are thankful for it every single day.

Then what does it take to become one of them? If most of the nation hasn't quite found the way to do it, there probably must be a specific way, steps to follow. Here is how to become grateful and thus bring satisfaction and contentment into your life.

- *Be aware*
  First, you need to become aware, not necessarily of the Way, especially if you're not ready for that, but be aware of the things you have. Contrary to what you may think, you do have many things you are probably unaware of. Think about the people in your life - family, friends, people who have helped you and supported you through hard times.

Remember every person in your life, even those who have insulted or betrayed you. And thank them for having the chance to learn the lesson they were meant to teach you. Every person we encounter on our way is meant to be there. They teach us something we can understand only if we are aware of that and are willing to learn from it.

Become aware of the things you have. Your home, job, places to go, clothes, technologies, the toys you played with, your books, and so on. Even if you don't live a luxurious life, you still have things that you use daily. Be aware of them, and don't take them for granted.

Be conscious of the things you do every day, which we don't even think of, and forget that they are a gift. Each day you eat a couple of times, most often food you love that tastes and looks so good, you take a shower whenever you want and use the amount of water you wish. You have electricity, and it allows you to do so many different things.

- *Appreciate the little things*
  To appreciate is to see that there is beauty in everything, notice little things and be thankful for them, and realize that what you have or do right now is amazing because others would give everything to have it.

Appreciation comes from within, because everything beautiful comes from in there. It is important for you to practice it until it becomes a habit, and once it does, everything will seem different to you, and you'll be much more content with life.

Appreciate things as they are now. Because they are perfect, all the circumstances, no matter how bad you consider them to be, all the people you meet, things you do, whatever you have or don't have, everything you experience and think of, is perfect just the way it is. And even if you'd like to change it, you first need to accept it as it is.

- *Slow your pace*
  We live in such a hurry that not only do we not notice the beautiful things surrounding us, but we also start to miss what matters - the people, events, and things that are right in front of our eyes. We rush through life, doing the daily tasks we consider important, working a job we can't stand, spending our free time in unconscious activities that only distract us from our purpose and journey (such activities are watching TV, browsing the net, and socializing online, using other technologies).

Sometimes you need to stop and take a breather. To stop means to take a moment now and then to look around, forget mundane things, problems, daily worries, selfish desires, fake goals, and current events, and focus on the essentials. Like your family, the things you love doing but never find time for, nature, opportunities.

- *Be Grateful*
  In a nutshell, you need to be thankful for everything around you every day. A good way to do it is to say it out loud. Make it a habit. Gratitude jars have become popular, and there's no reason why you can't try them out. It's a simple practice that includes writing down things you should be grateful for and putting them in a jar. Soon it will be full of

notes and you'll realize how many reasons you have in your life to be happy.

Another way is to make it a part of your morning or evening routine. Every day before bed or right after you get up, say everything you're grateful for in the mirror in the bathroom out loud. Try to feel excited about having it, smile, breathe deeply, and fill yourself with appreciation.

You can also put sticky notes in different places in your house. This way, you'll remind yourself of a thing to be grateful for whenever you enter a room. Keep a gratitude journal. Write down everything that happens to you for which you are grateful.

Choose the way that works best for you. And don't forget to enjoy the whole process. Becoming grateful is a big step in your personal development process and can work wonders. It will also have a positive influence on every other aspect of your life.

The final goal is to become mindful of everything you do, to do it with joy and excitement. It's time to be thankful and happy wherever you are.

Part III

THE HARMONY
OF BODY AND SPIRIT

Chapter One

INNER PEACE

L earning to protect body and mind, closing the door to the noise outside, helps us to recognize the importance that the spirit has in our life. We are not made of reason alone and even less of matter; our spiritual part, if nourished and developed, forms a solid ground on which to grow certainties.

To find ways and solve problems, the school teaches us from an early age how to use reason, helping us to develop our rational system. While this method penalizes emotions, it still seems the best way to prepare future generations.

But when we have to make an important decision, what do we make reason or heart prevail? Reflecting calmly, to better understand if it is an opportunity or something else, would be the best way to face important decisions, but finding moments of tranquility is increasingly difficult, because our thoughts are constantly interrupted by the noises of external confusion that they confuse and disorient us, postponing what we have to do.

Learning to protect body and spirit, closing the door to the noise outside, helps us to recognize the importance that the spirit has in our life. We are not made of reason alone and even less of matter; our spiritual part, if nourished and developed, forms a solid ground on which to grow certainties. To protect our spirit, we must take care of it as the gardener does with his garden, keeping it alive and luxuriant. Pauses of silent prayer or meditation make the flowers of awareness bloom and the branches of intuition grow that help us see the path to take.

In this sense, spirituality is also a practical technique for annihilating stress and daily fears that open the doors to many ailments that are harmful to our health. Spirituality helps us increase our focus, allowing us to give our best during decision making and making us more empathetic with others.

It also helps to achieve a deeper inner peace, transforming many negative beliefs with simple truths. Permanent physical ailments heal because the quality of life improves, we are more centered and objective, perceiving an inner wisdom that does not come from simple knowledge. By consolidating this lifestyle, it replaces uncertainties and anxieties with greater balance and consequent emotional stability which at the same time favors the body and mind. For some, they prefer to call it, 'inner peace.'

But then, isn't it all talk and nothing more?

Without mincing words, inner peace is not easy to find these days. The hectic pace of life we lead makes us stressful because we don't have the time we wish we had for ourselves.

There comes a time when we need to stop, put an end to unnecessary worries, and embark on the search for our inner peace.

Achieving inner peace means having a feeling of well-being, of happiness, which envelops us in immense tranquility.

It is about making a special connection with ourselves, making a connection between our body and spirit, as well as with the world around us, to be able to perceive details that we did not have, not aware of it before and, at the same time, to appreciate them.

In this state, we manage to isolate our mind: any fear, worry, negative thought or feeling that might bother us will be beyond our reach.

The benefits that come with inner peace
Let's focus on our goals.

Spirituality makes us more aware of what we want to achieve. If we know what our goals are and know exactly what we want, we will focus on achieving those goals.

a. *Avoid bad habits*
   By making a spiritual connection with ourselves and the world around us, we learn to differentiate between what is good and what is bad for us and for others. It will help us change our bad habits.

b. *The way to happiness*
   Inner peace allows us to channel our energy towards the positive aspects of our life, towards what makes us feel good. It will help us to be happier.

c. *Reduce stress*
   When we achieve spirituality, we learn to put aside all our concerns, which increases our level of psychological

well-being. As a result, all the accumulated stress will begin to disappear.

Is this then, a strife toward perfection?
"Perfection is not attainable, but if we aim for perfection, we can achieve excellence." - Vince Lombardi.

Despite all the drawbacks associated with possibility to turn perfectionism into a force without it compromising your health or your life in general? But then, it is possible.

For this, read these 8 tips that will help you find a harmonious and balanced life.

- *Be a balanced perfectionist, not neurotic*
  Perfectionism can be quite a healthy trait. Problems only appear when we live it to the extreme.

The vast majority of the problems exposed among the negative aspects of perfectionism, are actually extreme and toxic forms of perfectionism. Perfectionists who do this are neurotic and let their accomplishments define who they are. They often feel a deep discomfort in front of their goals and the future seems rather gloomy to them.

They always aim higher, to the detriment of everything, whether it is their relationships or their personal health. Unfortunately, this form of perfectionism is glorified in the media, where the focus is on the end result and not the sacrifices that led to the development of some innovation, or the achievement of a feat.

On the other hand, there is healthy perfectionism. This allows you to stay motivated while constantly seeking to improve. It does not focus on failures, but allows you to stay focused on the end goal.

By discovering the difference between these two forms of perfectionism, the healthy form and the neurotic form, you will be able to recognize the times when you slip into the dark side of perfectionism and moderate your behavior.

For this, let's move from perfectionism to optimalism and adopt the behavior accordingly.

- *Stop thinking in all-or-nothing mode*
  The "all-or-nothing" mentality is a big deal with perfectionists. Perfectionists have a very binary outlook on life. For them, it is either "White" or "Black", "All" or "Nothing", "Success" or "Fail", "Complete all" or "Start nothing".

Yet such a thought is self-defeating or at best, unreal. In the real world, no one achieves success without hiccups or failures. No athlete wins a competition without going to the trouble of training. No entrepreneur succeeds without first failing in some way or another.

And no one has produced great achievements without struggling with their tools, and without producing infamous drafts along the way. In reality, everything follows a progression, the all-or-nothing does not exist.

In Silicon Valley, there are thousands of companies including large multinationals like Facebook, Apple and Google who are encouraging failure. Countless successful entrepreneurs share the stories of their failures. There is even an annual conference called "Failcon" which encourages people to come to terms with their failures.

This is because they see failure as part of success, and by failing quickly you quickly learn what work, what doesn't, and grow from there.

Therefore, get rid of this all-or-nothing state of mind. When you think in all-or-nothing, what you get is more or less nothing-or-nothing. Allow yourself to do things incomplete, imperfect, and imprecise. Only then will you be able to progress in achieving your goal. Focus on recording your progress every step of the way, and use experimentation and failure lavishly, as this is the surest way to guarantee your future success.

- *Use the Pareto Principle*
  The mind of the perfectionist is a complex labyrinth. He is able to absorb large amounts of information, analyze details, and establish elaborate procedures for each task.

At the same time, you need to be careful not to fall into the vicious cycle of perfectionism, that is, the ability to drown yourself in countless information and parameters. Because a perfectionist is detail-oriented and able to store up mountains of information, this often prevents them from taking action.

For them, everything is important and everything must be done. In the end, they end up overwhelmed by the magnitude of what there is to accomplish. Some perfectionists procrastinate, others get stuck in analytical paralysis. Some give up, while others spend a lot of time just doing the most basic tasks.

Do you also tend to set yourself an extremely high bar for every task you do? Unfortunately, this expected level of quality often puts a damper on you, to the point where it prevents you from moving on. If so, here are some questions for you:

1. What are you trying to accomplish?
2. Who are the people who have succeeded in achieving this goal, or who tend to achieve it excellently today? What did they do to be successful?
3. Based on your answers to question 2, what details are you obsessed with ... Are they critical to the success of your goal? If not, is it time to put them aside (or reduce your investment on them)?

Focus on the 80/20 law and identify the few factors that are helping you the most in moving towards your goal. Beware of the law of diminishing returns, which occurs when you try to perfect every detail, especially those that have no influence on what you are trying to accomplish.

Chapter Two

HARMONY WITH ONESELF

We need to know that not everything is black and white, but that there is a whole range of grays. We have to accept that there are, and there will be, situations and experiences that we cannot control that will cause us to feel negative emotions, which are inevitably a part of our life. Achieving inner peace is synonymous with balance. There is no doubt that there will be unnecessary burdens that we can let go of, but we have to learn to deal with many others in our daily lives. That is why we must learn to balance our life, so that the mind stops fighting and ends up finding complete peace.

- **Simplify, you will conquer**
  We often complicate our lives and, as much as we find it hard to admit, it's up to us to make the most of every moment.

  If we reset our mind and let it get rid of unnecessary ideas and negative thoughts, then we can focus on our zest for life. By simplifying things, we will achieve inner peace, then we will be happier.

- **Listen to your inner self**
  With all these worries and thoughts flooding our minds, it is very difficult to talk to yourself. To be able to penetrate deep inside, we need a lot of calm, a silence that allows us to coexist with our own loneliness.

Listening to yourself in order to live in harmony with yourself is essential. If you don't listen to yourself, who will? Indeed, listening to your body, your mind and your emotions, you are the only one who has this super power:

The body is through ailments, bodily sensations, the 5 senses.

The mind by the thoughts and the fluidity of the information that we receive which naturally influences the mental load.

Emotions are manifested to guide us in our satisfactions, our choices and indicate to us if we are on our right track. Listening to yourself is also being anxious to respond to your needs, which are reflected in your emotions.

So listening to yourself means paying attention to what's going on inside you. A pleasant feeling symbolizes that all is well, a feeling of unease signals that something is not right for you. Finally, listening to yourself means being in agreement with your values, your desires, your personality and your aspirations.

In addition, it is a question of responding according to oneself and not according to what others expect (in an effective or supposed way). It is daring to know how to say "no" or to position oneself even though that would not suit everyone. Listening to them means trusting yourself and following your intuition, opinion and moods in order to live fully in harmony with yourself.

We have to learn to let ourselves go so that we know what our real internal concerns are. With a lot of patience and by slowing down our breathing, we can gradually achieve inner peace.

- **Keep the critics out of your life**
  Empathy is fundamental to moving forward on the path of inner peace. We have to put ourselves in other people's shoes.

Negative criticism towards others and ourselves makes us uncomfortable, it hurts both the recipient and the sender.

Get to know yourself. This process is not easy. In particular knowing that we are beings who evolve and we adapt to each age, to each event and each experience that arise. Some people will get to know each other while others will go through their lives without even thinking about it. It depends on our personality and our life course.

Knowing yourself means being aware of your strengths and resources as well as your weaknesses and limitations. Knowing yourself involves knowing what you want, what you aspire to and what you don't or no longer want. It is knowing your needs, your emotions, your capacities, your talents. It is also accepting his past, his good as well as his bad experiences, his relations, his ruptures, his personal/family/school/professional journey!

In addition, it is also about knowing its qualities and its faults. Even if some people advocate that we have the qualities of our faults and the faults of our qualities, it is nonetheless to be aware of who we are in our most beautiful imperfection is a source of well-being because a source of progress! When we know each other we know who we are, what we are worth and what direction to take for our future.

We must learn to see the positive side of things and to avoid all negative thinking, including criticism. The further we remove criticism from our life, the closer we will come to inner peace. We provide more details of this in the subsequent pages of this chapter.

- **The importance of meditation and reflection**
  To achieve inner peace, it is essential to calm our mind. For this the ideal is to carry out meditation exercises, which will help us to face the daily life better, with a more relaxed mind.

We have within us the capacities to know if what we are experiencing is good or not for us. It is possible for us to make choices, to remain in these choices or to modify them. We can't go back but we can always adjust to stay true to our own path. It is a wealth that we all have, regardless of the experience: we all have the choice and understanding each other allows us to experience them in harmony with oneself. It is very important for his well-being.

This power involves our ability to also understand our emotions, identify them and understand their signal. It is knowing the meaning that we put behind our actions, our ideas, our changes and our difficulties. Highlight our values and principles in our general behavior.

Understanding oneself includes the relationships we have, those we build and strengthen, but also those that we break or avoid. It is therefore to understand our expectations and our aspirations in the bonds that we form, in all areas: love, family, professional, friendly and social.

You should devote part of the day to regaining tranquility through meditation. In this way, our body and mind will be more predisposed to reflect and find the long-awaited inner peace.

In full consciousness, accept your strengths and your flaws, your qualities and your faults, your positive and negative emotions, etc. Everything that constitutes you and that makes you a unique and exceptional being! Living in harmony with yourself goes through this step! It is about respecting yourself in your entirety in order to achieve feelings of well-being and satisfaction.

Accepting yourself implies that you assume yourself as you are. It's knowing yourself, understanding yourself and not being afraid of it! Not afraid of not being accepted or being judged or criticized and fully asserting yourself in all awareness of who you are. It is possible for this to change vocabulary ("I am sensitive to injustice" for example rather than "I am angry", or "I have the character that I have" instead of "I have bad feelings character" - anyway what does "having a bad temper mean ??), change your attitude (no longer devalue yourself or fall into a box), change your view of things (practice positive communication) and work on your emotions negative social (such as shame).

- **You have to be thankful that you are well born**
  Recognizing life and all the positive things around us is fundamental to finding the path to inner peace. It helps us to be happier and to achieve balance.

There is always something to be thankful for, even if sometimes it is hard to believe it. When we reduce our complaints about what we don't have and begin to be grateful for what we have, we will regain our internal balance.

You have to love yourself. is to cherish yourself, to take care of yourself as a close friend or a member of your family. It's loving who you are and what you have. To love oneself is to adore what makes us up in our finest flaws.

We are indeed different: be it tall, short, fat, skinny, white, blue, black, neon or glitter, what does it matter? We are human! With our qualities, our faults, our experience, our family history, our desires, our dreams, etc. Everything that constitutes us makes us rich internally, to become aware of it with gratitude and benevolence: it is to love oneself. You really think you can live in harmony with yourself without loving yourself first?

To accept oneself is to accept this difference in a positive light. It is not because we do not think like everyone else, that we do not find ourselves in our place, that we do not fit "the mold" that it is a bad thing. The greatest geniuses of this world have often been "different", yet they have marked history.

We all make mistakes, no one is perfect and fortunately! This is what allows us to move forward and tend towards a "better", towards a change in order to love each other even more. Noticing who we have become despite the pitfalls and obstacles or even failures, isn't that self-love? Tolerance and mercy towards us?

To love yourself is to accept yourself fully with the best possible compassion and care. And it is by learning to love ourselves that it is possible for us to love others "healthily" (without emotional dependence, excessive jealousy, fear of abandonment or rejection, etc.) and to build relationships with all kinds that are fulfilling.

When you love yourself, it is easier to love others. So there is no question of accepting toxic and devaluing relationships. Or not to accept violence, mistreatment; whether physical, mental or emotional. We only seek to build and move forward with positivity and serenity in the Love of oneself, others and its environment.

Generosity, giving without receiving anything in return, is linked to gratitude. We must move away from selfishness to come closer to peace and serenity.

- **The power of forgiveness**
  The act of forgiving and asking for forgiveness has a therapeutic effect which is fundamental to achieving

spiritual peace. Through forgiveness, we trade destructive behaviors towards the person who hurt us for constructive behaviors.

Forgiveness is also, for ourselves, probably the most difficult thing to give. It is precisely at this stage that we must insist on achieving inner calm.

The act of forgiveness is complex because it is not an isolated moment, on the contrary. It is an ongoing process that can be deepened and completed over time.

Chapter Three

CONNECTION BETWEEN THE BODY AND SPIRIT

As established in the previous chapter, the body is composed of flesh and bones. It is a physical container that houses the spirit, while the spirit is your state of consciousness. It is the ability to accept changes (feelings, thoughts, actions, and behavior) in your life.

Understanding The Connection Between The Body And Spirit

Man is always searching for happiness and, as such, pursues mundane things to fulfill their thoughts or consciousness. For instance, due to the desire as humans to be loved, valued, and needed, some people participate in social media activities by posting pictures and engaging in contests. Doing this helps them feel noticed and validated as they receive recognition from strangers that fool them into thinking they are loved and accepted.

> *Great Virtue of practice is with the Way*
> *The Way cannot be touched or captured*
> *It cannot be felt or captured*

But there's an image inside
It cannot be supposed or captured
But there is a category inside14
The Way is dim
But inside has substance
This substance is genuine
Which contains belief
From the primitive to the present
The Way is eternal
The Way is the creation
How do we know that Way is the root of all creatures?
Chapter 21 -The Book of Ethics

Receiving recognition may satisfy that craving for validation for a short while. One may even be happy for a while; however, as the world moves on to the next exciting thing, the feelings of dissatisfaction with oneself returns. It is an insatiable feeling that is due to the entire state of one's mind. In life, the search for happiness is in the Way-which is Spiritual Enlightenment. If you were wondering, Yes, the body and spirit can be harmonized.

The Way does not act
But nothing is not done
If the king notices this
Then everything will change itself
If one wants to do
Be simple and rustic
Be invisible without desire
When there is no desire, then you will be undisturbed
This is the path to self-healing.
Chapter 37- The Book of Ethics

The body and spirit are interrelated, closely connected, and reciprocal in action. It simply means the issues of life steams from within. As understood from the story, a change in heart was responsible for the difference in appearance. Spiritual strength/enlightenment yields physical well-being. To find true happiness, it is necessary to be in a state of spiritual enlightenment - The Way.

To a school of thought, the body is a hindrance in living purposefully and finding happiness. Why? The body is perceived as a lowly nature, full of sin, evil, and actions contrary to our desire. Looking at the life of a kleptomaniac, these individuals pick petty items too ridiculous to be stolen by the will of their bodies. How can the body move without the permission of the spirit? The act of theft is carried out in a state of unconsciousness. Perhaps, could it be an imbalance in the spiritual enlightenment needed for the body to vibrate at a specific frequency? Cases like these and more make it difficult for one to understand the balance between spirit and body.

Nevertheless, being a physical being does not imply evil and sin. The purpose of the body is to serve the spirit. The relationship between the two elements is beautiful. Interestingly, the spirit cannot be made perfect without the body. Only with the body can the spirit find purpose.

What does this mean?

> *People with profound Virtue like babies*
> *Bees and snakes cannot spit poisonous nibs*
> *Wild beasts cannot grab*
> *Birds can't peck*

Soft bones and weak tendons
But hold firm
Don't know how to have sexual intercourse between men and
women
But perfect vitality is living in abundance
Screaming all day but not hoarse
That is called Harmony
Knowing the Harmony is invariant
Knowing invariants is bright
Greed is catastrophe
Being greedy is not Harmony
Disharmony is the opposite of the Way
The opposite of the Way is soon destroyed.
Chapter 55 – The Book of Ethics

It simply means:
When one is indeed in the Way, Harmony is achieved. Being in a state of consciousness is a character only possible with a body. As much as the spirit's will wants to be expressed, it is limited to a living body. That is to say, the body without the spirit is dead. Wow! What harmonization. The body, spirit relationship is directly proportional to each other, whereby the body's functioning is dependent on the spirit, vice-versa.

The correlation between the spirit and body can be said thus: The purpose of our spiritual enlightenment is to bring Harmony through our body. Our spiritual strength influences physical well-being. Our thoughts and feelings trace their source from within and translate into physical experiences, which become our actions and behavior.

Feel opposed, suffocated, excited, satisfied, valued, etc., is the inter-relationship between spirit and body. Our noble feelings are expressed in the physique.

Victor Hugo said, "No external grace is complete unless vivified by internal beauty."

Let's take into cognizance an account of a trip you embarked on with your family to a resort center. On your arrival, you had a glance at the environment. It was picturesque, serene, scenic, and a sight to behold. However, after you showered and had lunch, with slow strides around the resort, you began to notice imperfections in the structure. Even though the flaws saw, the peace, calm, good energy you felt at your arrival was not lost. That is true beauty springing from a state of Harmony. True beauty is the purity, radiance, Harmony, light that emanates from a person's inner light, which actualizes in the bodily form.

After an accident made him blind, French writer Jacques felt like the world had come crashing down against him. However, as he journeyed in life, he saw the light never seen throughout the days; his organs of sight were functional, and he concluded, "To be blind meant not to see but, I saw." The testimony of this young man and others who have lost their sense of sight, perception, or one thing or the other is an eye-opener that indeed, spiritual enlightenment is what brings balance and harmony to our body; what you see within translates without.

Do not go out but know the world
Do not look out the window but see the Way
The more one goes, the less one knows
So, a sage does not go out but knows
Do not only look but see
Do not only do but accomplish.
Chapter 47 – The Book of Ethics

Your manner and Way of life affect balance. One needs to be careful of the physical image he paints to the world. Live a life that portrays your spiritual enlightenment to yield proper balance. As you notice imbalance and lack of Harmony, it is proof that you lack enlightenment and you will need to work on this.

Chapter Four

BALANCE AND HARMONY

M any of us wonder about the essence of harmony between the body, spirit, and soul. The foundational pillars of harmonious life are based on these components. The body and spirit have to be in constant relationship and balance to attain harmony. The energy generated within our inner state of consciousness, the actions that this energy produces outward to the seeing of others, and the channeling of power from the cosmos (the Earth and its components) have to be perfected as one sound, united together to sustain a peaceful life.

We have experienced several situations in life that are easily relatable to understand what not living in harmony entails. Some examples are:

1. In most cases, we find ourselves thinking, overworking, and beating ourselves up concerning adverse events that happened in our lives than the good times we had. For instance, if you are offered a position, or you relocate to a new school, nation, etc., your initial response to this situation will be negative. You think of how difficult it is to

cope, feeling alone or left out, the hardships, contrary to how that circumstance will profit you greatly. If we are sincere with ourselves, we discover that we are designed to be full of negatives. Sadly, this is interpreted as your spirit (state of consciousness) not being in harmony with itself.

2. Using the body as an example, what we experience all comes down to your self-perception. Just as a lot of our young ones face today, the craze to have an image everyone appreciates on social media is on a high. However, suppose we confront most of them to know how they see themselves when they look at the mirror or, better still, do a practical test of each one facing the mirror and telling us whose image they see reflecting. In that case, it will amaze you to know that a significant percentage of those smiling, gorgeous, cute, well-dressed ladies and gentlemen do not see advancement into what they aspire to become or beauty in themselves. It only means you are not in harmony with your body.

3. Regarding the spirit, if you look carefully, some of your neighbors, friends, or acquaintances who are spiritually enlightened have a defined way of life. One notable thing about them is the desire to learn, being knowledgeable, and the ease they offer the knowledge gained over time. Either way, a life of giving and receiving is their culture. In plain terms, they are not inflexible, living in a box; they have stretched their body and spirits beyond and grown drastically by their and others' experiences and knowledge.

Ponder on these questions: do you believe you understand everything? Do you show interest in learning anything that arouses your curiosity? Do you judge the source of what you are learning? After your honest evaluation of these questions and your answer to any is NO, it is disheartening that you are not in harmony with your body and spirit.

What is Harmony?

Harmony is a powerful Chinese expression describing the chase for balance between a man, his atmosphere, people, and spirit. The concept of harmony is as such wise and philosophical.

Harmony exudes diversity first, then balance. It is how a lot is combined with being balanced. When diverse thoughts, concepts, colors, and actions are balanced, it produces a harmonious event. For example, imagine a group of persons singing in the same tone. What do you see? Beautiful singing without melody or richness. However, when other techniques are added to the singing group, we experience a rich, refined blend of tones producing a harmonized sound. Now, the various styles we heard singing came together to create a balanced effect. This is the theory of harmonization.

Fundamentals of Harmony

The theory of harmonization exists because of some particular truths, which makes for Its foundation and strengthens its convictions.

1. **Yin-Yang Oneness:** Taoism is greatly influenced by the Chinese theory of Yin and Yang opposites. Yin is dark, and Yang is light. They are both intertwined and connected, representing balance and harmony. When your yin and yang are in harmony, it is possible to prolong your life, and otherwise, your life is shortened and susceptible to diseases. Hence, harmony is based on the yin-yang oneness.

You need to understand the 'oneness' principle because you are part of it. To attain this level of oneness, a rich connection with nature, the earth, and its elements are required. By learning to be an observer of nature, you take note of its rhythm and interconnection amongst all elements. You must become like water.

1. **Wei-wu-Wei:** This means swimming with the current, stooping in to conquer, etc. It is the flow that makes it possible for an individual to achieve harmony with all things. Wei-Wu-Wei means to follow or without acting on, allowing things to be within nature. It is not passive or living to chance. It is flowing with Earth (nature) as it flows with Heaven and feedback of Heaven as Tao (nature). Just as it rains, Heaven and Earth are seen uniting. The showers that fall upon the Earth are responded to naturally by humans without a command or instruction. That is Wei Wu Wei; Flowing freely with nature as it communicates with us.

2. **Water characteristics:** In the Book of Ethics by Lao Tzu, water was used severally to communicate the water features of Taoism. Water moves swiftly and is always serving others, humble, transparent, etc. This is therefore understood as the water characteristic of Tao. The main features that make up the water characters include:

A. Altruism is the ability to pour yourself, serve others entirely without any form of expectation. Water is an essential need of life that all organisms depend on for survival and habitation for another. Taoists should be just like water.

B. Modesty and Humility; As rightly explained, water maintains a low profile after its great acts of service. If we all are altruistic, possessing the heart of service and humility, the numerous conflicts we face in the world would drastically reduce. The Way teaches a nature that does not show off but is ready to learn and remain low amidst the applause of men.

Modesty and humility are virtues that help a man harmonize with himself, others, and influential leaders. Like the sea that births numerous streams and rivers, humility makes a leader accept the visions of others as theirs and work towards achieving them. Such people attract others to themselves and work in unity for one purpose.

C. Adaptability and flexibility; Water can take the shape/ size of any container. Humans are also known to be able to adapt to any situation. However, we do not see this in full expression. Adaptability is a skill required for exceptional leadership; the ability to handle any situation. Also, rigidity hinders you from flowing freely with nature. To be in a harmonious state, you have to be flexible.

D. Transparency and Clarity; When an individual is honest and transparent in his ways, they are said to be a person of integrity. If no one makes water unclean, it remains fine. Yet, it is made clean by allowing the impurities to settle. Likewise, as humans, external factors tend to make us muddy and unclean, which differs from our true nature.

E. Soft but persistent; Gentle but powerful; Taoism teaches us to be soft in embracing the uniqueness of others yet constant in flowing freely with nature. Water is a subtle yet powerful tool whose traits should be emulated. What about the negative features of water, you ask? Whenever Yin and Yang are not in harmony, disasters like floods and water-related disasters occur solely due to external factors (acts of man).

4. **Love for peace:** Lao Tzu- the founder of Taoism, lived in an ancient time of the Zhou Dynasty when people and states were at war with each other. His utter dislike for violence made him resign as a historian in the Imperial city to live as a hermit on the mountain. In opposition to war and its likes, he has been an advocate of peace from the onset.

    Taoism is firmly against acts that lead to the detraction of lives and properties. As such, harmony boasts peaceful living.

5. **Tolerance and appreciating differences:** Openness and tolerance are critical aspects of Taoism that foster harmony with nature and other individuals. The world is a complicated place; being open and tolerant is necessary to harmonize with nature and one another. It is against The Way to aspire to be like someone else. Everyone is created uniquely with differences, and that is what brings harmony to our world.

Harmony, therefore, means tolerating, understanding, and appreciating human differences.

Balance in the Body and Spirit

Meditation and spiritual enlightenment are essential in obtaining inner harmony. Physical harmony is dependent on good health. A healthy body is not just fit or built but in tune with the spiritual vibrations from within and responds accordingly. Sometimes, the body's immune system gets weak, and we fall ill. During those moments, the body does all it can to restore balance and fight. You are expected to help your body maintain that balance by taking medications, eating the proper diet, taking fluids frequently, etc.

Also, when you conform to the consciousness of the spirit by maintaining inner beauty, frequency, and vibe in a manner that only allows the inflow of pure/godly thoughts, it is a state of spiritual balance.

According to Chinese philosophy and medicine, yin and yang (female - moon and male - sun attributes) need to be in harmony for all life to flow through it. Fill the heart (spirit) with harmony and balance. It will lengthen life - Guan Zi. The yin and yang symbol mean homeostasis and self-maintenance; it brings to remembrance the importance of balance.

A skilled plant is difficult to eradicate
A skilled grasp is difficult to slip
Virtue will be honored from generation to generation
By fixing Virtue in oneself, Virtue will be real
By fixing Virtue in the house, Virtue will have redundancy
By fixing Virtue in the village, Virtue will grow
By fixing Virtue in the country, Virtue will be in abundance
By fixing Virtue in the world, Virtue will be everywhere

So, by oneself that considers others
By one's house that considers other houses
By one's village that considers other villages
By one's nation that considers other nations
By one's people that consider other people
How do we know what people are? Thanks for that!
Chapter 54 – The Book of Ethics

Balance versus Harmony

Balance is the way humans behave. An average person is to act in a balanced, law-abiding manner concerning the environment. Normalcy is a static form that humans find hard to relate to because they are dynamic.

Unlike balance, harmony is not static; that is, fixed in a place. It is a flexible term that connotes locomotion. Every individual is a product of his decisions, passions, and thoughts, not his circumstances. The way you think has a significant role to play in your reaction or response to events. Situations do not make men instead; men make situations, especially if the state of consciousness is not beclouded.

Hence, finding balance is objective and rational, while harmony is subjective and visceral. Harmony is a better concept than balance due to the ease of being flexible and adaptable.

It is easier to maintain harmony than achieve balance. When we feel joy, insight, wisdom, euphoria, they are subjective ideals making it more practical for internal harmony to be sought.

Harmony is felt when we accept our nature, who we are present. It is a perception of both positives and negatives towards our identity. What you consider your:

- Strengths and weaknesses
- Achievements and failures
- Talents and defects, etc.

You build a harmonious nature when you accept yourself wholly, flaws and all. The challenges that self-rejection causes are more significant than we can imagine; low self-esteem, personality disorders, thieves, verbally and physically abusive individuals, panic disorders, and bullying. It is difficult not to feel wronged concerning our limitations. However, that is what makes us unique. They are the yin and yang tones, expressions that join together to form harmony.

Light and darkness in Christianity is a group of morals. Light is seen as being morally upright, worthy of emulation, while darkness is evil, to be defeated.

Make it all empty
Keep your mind calm
All species born also pass away
Then they go back to the original source12
Returning to the origin is stillness
It is according to the law of nature
The natural law is immutable
Knowing the circulation of heaven and Earth is lucid
No knowing the circulation of heaven and Earth is dark
Knowing the circulation is lucid

By being lucid, then the soul is exuberant
By being exuberant, then the soul behaves fairly
Fairness is everywhere
Everywhere is suitable with nature
What is suitable with nature is suitable with the Way
Being one with the Way is the accurate Way
Even when the body dies, the Way remains.
Chapter 16 – The Book of Ethics

However, the Taoist approach states that darkness is a natural flow and rhythm of the universe and should not be overcome. Achieving balance from the Taoist view aligns yourself with the cosmos (world) and a life of harmony with nature resulting from the belief in natural order or The Way.

The Way is the eternal breath
The Way is a woman
The woman is the mother of the beginning stage
The mother's gateway is the root of heaven and Earth
Like a veil very hard to see
Using the Way will never dry out.
Chapter 6 – The Book of Ethics

How to Achieve a Balanced Life

A balanced life is paramount for oneness and harmonious living in society. The following are methods to achieving a balanced life:

1. *Be objective in your approach*
   As the Way, there is no discrimination between light and dark, good and evil. It would be best if you accepted everything and everyone. The perspective of good and evil

must be blocked from your mind, paying no attention to personal preference. Defining circumstances, individuals, and others in our environment cause conflict.

Examples:
If you see modesty as good, you will most likely paint whatever is perceived as indecent to you as bad.

A lady who greets persons is homely and respectful; ladies who do contrary to that are disrespectful and cannot manage a home.

2. *Accept the natural course of life than defining its qualities*
   A lot of us like to think things through thoroughly. Why ponder over things again and again when you certainly have no control over the situation. It is healthier and beneficial not to try to make sense out of it. Giving meaning to a natural progression only makes the process painful.

3. *Move on to the past or think of the future.* Live your life in the now, making wise use of what life offers to you.
   The past is past; it is behind, and you cannot turn the hands of time. Stop sulking and enjoy the flow brought to your doorsteps.

Examples:
You are at the beach, unwinding and sipping a cold drink with the provision of a coconut shade to obstruct the sunlight rays and keep you cool. But it begins to rain suddenly. Usually, this unforeseen circumstance should ruin your mood; however,

instead of feeling miserable, dance in the rain and enjoy the moment.

4. *Allow the universe to introduce your school of thought*
   Your ideologies are not forcefully passed worldwide. At this age, everyone has something to say, even when it's sensible or not. They crave relevance, and their influence is overwhelming. There is an excellent population of people who claim to be teachers/scholars. The only thing they do is give out advice, teachings, information without a desire to listen to another's perspective.

Benefits of Maintaining a balanced Lifestyle

- *It alleviates stress* - by taking time to exhale and inhale, it slows down your pace, allows you to relax and be more objective in your decisions.
- *It enhances your mood* - the noise that comes from the cares and worries of this life will most likely weigh you down. However, taking breathing exercises will help you brighten up.
- *It aids in boosting energy* - energy is the ability to do work. The balance, therefore, helps in channeling the flow of energy to the right places for productivity.
- *It betters your state of mind* - we are in constant war with our minds, affecting the quality of our inner state without our conscious knowledge.
- *It increases longevity and reduces aging* - the simplicity of balance takes away stress, bodily fatigue. Aging is caused by numerous stressors that take a toll on the physique. Remember, our inner consciousness produces our physical

form. Therefore a troubled inner state will yield a troubled and worn-out physical form.

- *It prevents health-related diseases* - the issues of life are from within. Too much of everything is bad for your health. You should take life step by step. Excess activities stimulate the production of body hormones resulting in a hard time for the body to pick up with it and maintain homeostasis.
- *It boosts your self-worth and confidence* - performing at maximum level is only possible when you maintain balance. Your words, steps, and even inactions exhume confidence.
- *It gives you an understanding of life* - In seeing life from a more straightforward angle, you realize there is no rush in life; you take things slowly and live in the moment!
- *It enables you to be selfless* - true satisfaction is obtained from helping others become better versions of themselves or providing the platform on which they can become empty individuals who pour themselves into humanity without expectations or commendations.
- You master how to handle life issues and challenges without affecting your inner state.
- You attract positive energy and abundance from the flow of life.

My sayings are simple to understand, simple to practice
But people do not understand
Therefore, people do not practice
My words have the root
My job is well-structured
Because people do not understand me
So, they don't know me
People who understand me are tiny

People who follow me are rare
So, the sage wears the rough cloth
But the heart embraces precious jewels.
Chapter 70 – The Book of Ethics

The Importance of Harmony in Life

Harmony is a spice of life that spurs togetherness among individuals and Nations. It is the capacity to handle different areas of our lives. Individual harmony must be attained to have a free flow of energy with nature. Hence, every individual must effectively cope and provide solutions for areas in our lives that seek to stress and frustrate our inner peace. Chinese culture takes harmonization seriously. Through harmony, people share their perspectives without conflicts.

The Importance of Peace in Life

For every human and even society, desiring a peaceful environment to thrive and succeed is essential. Violence affects the harmony and balance of society. To live a balanced life, our inner peace should be undisturbed to channel energy flow properly. We have to understand situations that cause disturbances and handle them, such as anger, fear, insecurity, etc. We appreciate and honor each other when we live in peace despite our religious, social, and cultural differences.

A peaceful person orchestrates harmony and maintains such relationships amongst others and society.

Peace and Harmony are interdependent and related. It is a fundamental necessity for living.

Living in harmony fosters community building and development. The power of Harmony amongst individuals cannot be under-emphasized. The crisis, wars, violence, hardships, and other mishaps in society result from individuals or groups of persons who refuse to understand the uniqueness of man forcefully desiring others to accept their way of life.

The mindset of peace and Harmony is endorsed by a healthy way of life as resolving conflicts, tolerance, adaptation, empathy, etc.

> *The perfect one is like water*
> *Water provides life for all things*
> *Without competing with anything*
> *Water lives where people hate*
> *Therefore, it can be compared with the Way*
> *Accommodation is humble*
> *Thinking is deep*
> *Treatment is forgiven*
> *Talking is genuine*
> *Assertiveness is fair*
> *Working is competent*
> *Action is timely*
> *When there's no contest, then there will be no mistakes.*
> *Chapter 8 – The Book of Ethics*

How to Live in Peace and Harmony

Since we have established the importance of peace and Harmony in our daily lives, we would look at some steps to take in achieving a peaceful and harmonious life:

- *Make time for yourself daily*
  Our present generation keeps us glued to social media, work, extracurricular activities, etc. With such trends and a

sense of busyness, it is easy to lose ourselves and get carried away by one thing or another. Creating a time for yourself to unwind and relax is something we need to balance yin and yang. A time for activities also requires a time to be still, calm, and flow with the energy within you. Do not forget, the imbalance in yin and yang causes diseases that shorten your lifespan.

- *Live your life intentionally each moment*
  Don't linger on memories. Instead, learn from your previous mistakes, apply the solutions to your present. Worrying about the future is futile. The decisions you make now will give you the future you desire.

- *Ensure that your choices and decisions are carefully thought of before making a move*
  Don't make decisions you will regret. As much as The Way advocates going with the flow of nature, it does not imply living your life to chance. An actual state of oneness would make you so harmonious that it extends to your outward appearance, which involves your actions. Actions are products of your decisions - a mental and physical balance yields productivity. Make sure the principles of the Way back your choices.

- *Think before reacting to situations*
  The Way is against violence and its acts. Making rash decisions has led to outbursts of anger, regretful decisions, death, wars, and so on. Hence, follow the Way of peace and harmony at all times. Flow with the equilibrium of your inner state.

- *Meditate*
  Meditation is a necessary means of attaining peace and harmony. It has been rightly discussed in the previous chapter. Meditative practices foster stillness and focus. This aids inner peace and harmony. Make sure to engage in reflective exercises, often even for 10-20 minutes daily.

- *Engage in selfless activities*
  By giving your time and effort to a worthy cause to harmonize the environment, society will assist you in living a peaceful life. Activities like global warming, giving to the needy, anti-pollution campaigns, etc. A faithful follower of the Way seeks to empty themselves for the betterment of nature. Engaging in such enhances your inner state of peace and balance.

- *Make sure to surround yourself with peaceful and harmonious people or things*
  Spending your time watching, reading, or listening to violent/disturbing content, including video games, will make you lose harmony. Get healthy materials that will help you attain harmony. When you have the right company around you, it helps to strengthen your faith and boosts harmonious living. The best company to keep are those who are on the same path as you.

Eliminate learning and worry less
What differentiates good and evil?
Why are we scared of what others are afraid of?
So immense, it is impossible to know.
Everyone is as cheerful as when enjoying a buffalo feast

Like spring on the hill
I am silent alone
Like an infant who cannot yet laugh
Hanging down, walking like a homeless person
People have become redundant
I am destitute alone
My mind is like a fool
How dumb!
People are all bright and sharp
My own is dark and dull
People like the ocean's waves
I do not know which way the wind is blowing
People are busy
My own boorish
I am different from people
I'm unlike other people
I trust in mother's milk to feed all species.
Chapter 20 – The Book of Ethics

Chapter Five

HOW TO GET FINANCIAL HARMONY

Greed, corruption, and envy seep into your heart when you do not live a harmonious life. The beauty of Harmony is in satisfaction. As humans, the tendency to get jealous and covetous of others is excellent. Most times, we feel bad when our counterparts have attained a height we are yet to reach. This is not the way.

Great Way spreads everywhere
It moves to the left and moves to the right
It is depended on everything
It creates without holding back
Work is accomplished, yet taking credit
The Way fosters all species without mastering
Without desire, it is called small
All species come back without mastering
And so are called great
In the end, the Way doesn't receive as marvelous itself
That is why it accomplished a great thing.
Chapter 34 – The Book of Ethics

Harmony regarding finances is achievable when you channel all the negative thoughts into the proper flow of life. Block the bad energy, check your heart, ponder on the reasons why you are stuck in a stagnant position, rather than envy, appreciate the people who have attained the height you desire.

The law of honor states that you attract what you celebrate. In appreciating your superiors and those at the same level as you, you channel the proper flow of energy to yourself.

Too much noise in our inner selves is responsible for the bad decisions we make. It is possible to live a humble, satisfied and appreciative life.

Often, life circumstances push us beyond limits exposing us to the imbalance that causes chaos. No man was born evil. The state of their consciousness and spiritual enlightenment was relatively poor that it could not contain their body; hence they made choices contrary to the Way.

Asides from the circumstances we are faced with, a specific career path we take pushes us towards internal Imbalance and chaos. Having a work and life balance is essential.

It is no doubt that you have heard of situations where rivalry in workplaces, government offices, marketplaces, etc., has pushed others into evil. The competition produces bad energy that leads to chaos and violence amongst us. People no longer see eye to eye; arguments, misunderstandings, threats, and even death become the order of the day.

Skilled walker leaves no footprints
Skilled talker does not miss words
A skilled mathematician does not need a comparison
Skillfully closed needs not locking
But no one can open it
Skillfully knotted needs not tied
But no one can remove it
Sage takes care of everyone
Not missing one
Sage takes care of everything
Nothing missing anything
That is called bright-hearted!
Who is a good person?
The teacher of the bad person
Who is the bad person?
Someone meant for the good person to teach
If the teacher is not respected
And the student does not love
Then there is confusion in talent
That is the pivotal point of the mystery.
Chapter 27 – The Book of Ethics

The path of Harmony is the solution to the chaos the world is facing. Our inner selves require this harmony to help us be at a state of equilibrium and peace. Satisfaction is harmony. A man who is content and satisfied with his resources is so blessed that life he issues have no hold on him. There is no room for hatred, mischief, lies, and all sorts.

Steps to take in achieving financial harmony

- Choose a career path you are satisfied with: The problem is satisfaction. Choosing a career path should not come from greed; instead, to help society and man at large. Making an impact and creating balance for a peaceful world is the responsibility of every man. If you are satisfied with yourself and what you do, no man will push you to the wall.

- Be peaceful with yourself and others: Yes! We want to be better and achieve greater heights. However, every man has time to attain a peak in life, finances, influence, and relevance. Be at peace, be diligent, and the right moment will come to you. If there is no peace in the world, even the height you hope to attain would be snatched from you.

- Practice meditation: Positive affirmations and hearing motivating speeches will translate to your spirit. Meditating daily shapes your thoughts and innermost desires. You are what you listen to. Take time to invest in your meditations. Ensure to have these solitary moments day and night

- Be vocal about appreciating others: Emptiness makes you reach out to others without restrain, pretense or pride. Relate with others because you want to know them genuinely, not for ulterior motives. Search your heart daily, think about what your innermost heart contains. Don't hide your true motives, it only takes a moment for your spirit to be known by all men.

The highly virtuous people do not pray for virtue;
they already have virtue
The lowly virtuous people want virtue, so they don't have virtue
The highly virtuous people do nothing
Yet nothing is undone

The lowly virtuous people always do
Yet many more things need to be done
The humane person works without letting the job go unfinished
The righteous person works, but the undone jobs are many
The polite person works, but no one responds
When the Way dies, the Virtue is born
When the Virtue dies, humanity is born
When humanity dies, the righteous is born
When the righteous die, the polite is born
Politeness is a shell of disloyalty
The clue of chaos
Using the mind to foresee flashes the Way
The clue of foolishness
Highly virtuous people live faithfully
They do not respect politeness
On the fruit, neither in the flower
One chooses this but leaves that.
Chapter 38 – The Book of Ethics

Chapter Six

HARMONY AND HEALTH

Health by the Way is based on allowing the Tao to flow with ease and maintaining the harmony of the universe. In previous times, health was defined as Harmony and balance. The purpose of the Way is to grasp nature and live in harmony with it through the understanding gained. When mental or physical ailments/illnesses occur, it just implies that harmony is lost in the inner state. The Way provides solutions to the world's current dilemma: balance, harmony, relaxation/peace, and moderation.

Since the way is directly in tune with nature, it is expected that the standard approach to health will require natural methods.

The following health care practices for Taoists are described:

1. **Palliative care** - For people in the Way, natural sources of alleviating pain are the most practical choice. If medication serves its aim of recalibrating the body's natural ability to function, drugs are not out of bounds. The flow of nature will take its course when treatment has stopped being responsive.

2. **Self-decisions and Patient's authority** - The family has a significant role in the end-of-life decisions for Taoists.

3. **Death and Beyond** - Death is Natural. However, Taoist believes that it does not cut ties between the dead and the living.

> *By keeping body and soul together*
> *Is it possible to keep them apart?*
> *Pay attention to breathe*
> *To be soft*
> *Can one become an infant?*
> *With spiritual cleansing*
> *Can the stain be gone?*
> *Love people and rule country*
> *The heaven gate opens and closes*
> *Through everything*
> *Can't we do anything?*
> *We are born and raised*
> *Instructions without possessions*
> *Made without merit*
> *Instruction without ruling*
> *Such is the root of the Way*
> *Chapter 10 – The Book of Ethics*

Lifestyle Practices for Longevity

1. *Live life fully*
   Life is lived to its fullest daily, as it is loaded with experiences and richness. This manner of living creates a means for one to be healthy, flexible, and robust. Pursuing means to elongate one's life artificially leads to critical shortenings of life. It is against the Way, which advocates a natural flow.

2. *Eat good meals*

The quality of life one expects to have is directly connected to the diet one takes. For the body to function correctly for a long time, you must eat a well-prepared, balanced and healthy diet. Eating a properly balanced diet is Key. A subtle reason many diets or nutrition is inadequate is that we refuse to change or upgrade our diet according to our respective bodies' needs. There is no particular meal that contains the essential and balanced nutrients required by the body. Instead, it is our responsibility to listen to our body's needs and offer vital mixtures to the body. Green tea, Cabbage, Yogurt, and Brown rice are foods of higher quality than others.

As a follower of the Way, the life cycle of the food we eat and its practices before its death, especially livestock, should be carefully considered before consumption. The Way teaches a habit of respecting food processing and intake with balance and moderation.

3. *Obey nature*

Our world is incredibly distracted; numerous goals to achieve, a lot of ideas to implement, a list of desires to accomplish, other factors trying to influence, compete and lead you with a belief system they consider higher than yours. You can never attain a long life with all these distracting sounds. However, bringing all sound together is advantageous; harmony gives you an edge over others because of the Way.

The Way advocates Nature. As you get older, you begin to walk with nature dutifully. Adulthood changes like menopause, reduced energy, loss of sight, etc., are not ignored but used for personal expansion.

4. *Exercise regularly*
Physical fitness is not optional. You have to keep your body in perfect condition and functioning. Qigong is an exercise practice that is beneficial to keep the body agile and in good shape. The fact that physical fitness is essential does not mean that you overwork yourself and overstretch your body. Dance through life; do not fight life or your body. None is the enemy - the Way.

5. *Attitude*
Treating your body as the opponent or a container that should be subjected at all costs limits your life. The rate at which you resist the world is directly proportional to the rate the world restricts you. This is already a lost battle because, in comparison with the world, which is bigger and larger, one entity is nothing and will be easily swallowed. Fighting back excessively would only wear you down. Are we saying don't fight back? Allow yourself to be tossed by any and everything? No, stand up for yourself but not against the world ruthlessly. It will wash you away.

The proper lifestyle of the Way is a good sense of humor, low stress, and a positive outlook.

6. *Have a spiritual practice*
Spiritual practice is a mixture of intentions with actions and the discovering of mysteries in life. It is highly advised to engage in spiritual activity to keep harmony between your mind and body as a boost, mind, and spirit. Think of this as the practice by which an individual discovers peace with nature.

A healthy, sound spiritual practice is a component of the Way. Many of the techniques are related to Shamanism. Everyone is expected to establish his practice. These practices are a source of inspiration for leading a lengthier happy life. There are diverse kinds of training based on philosophy, science, religion, magic, etc. One thing, however, that strikes a balance amongst these numerous views is the acceptance of the Way.

7. Avoid addiction

The Way describes addiction as a redefinition of the space with an external factor to nature while living is to be yourself. Life is a push, and the struggles we encounter are a means to sharpen us. Usually, addictions seem like a means to make life easier, which is false . It is a dead-end.

Be open to humiliation
What does "be open to humiliation" mean?
Accept bad luck like its human destiny
Reception is not important
Do not worry about loss or gain
This is called "be open to humiliation."
What does "accept bad luck like it is human destiny" mean?
Bad luck comes from one's body
If not, where does that bad fortune come from?
Be precious to one's body
As people believe one's body is everything
Love this world like one's body
Then one can fulfill everything.
Chapter 13 – The Book of Ethics

Chapter Seven

LIVING A BALANCED LIFE

A balanced life is not restricted to a certain way. There are numerous ways for you to live a balanced life. The ball is in your court; it always has! The simplest way to be balanced is by harmonizing your body and spirit. Keep in mind that the goal of this is to live in harmony, thereby attracting plenty.

Our top goal in this life is to live in harmony with ourselves (body and spirit) and everything in our environment. Harmony is the pathway to balance. Balance yields peace and abundance.

If you are on a path to attain balance, your progress is measured based on your internal flow. When we obstruct a particular flow in our body, it will sprout in a way spiritual, social, or otherwise. Imbalance is caused by the inevitable challenges in life that confront us and hinder our growth. Taoist are of the school of thought that when people apply the concept of yin and yang, they will realize that just as the symbols preach harmony and balance, the interlocking spirals show that life is an ever-changing passage. Hence both light and dark are necessary for balance.

Affirming that you have yin and yang moments that have shaped you into who you are is not all to balance. The functionality of life of credit comes with striking an understanding between these phases.

Living a balanced life is possible by having an objective approach to life. You must be capable of embracing every person without prejudice.

Stillness is easy to grasp
Formlessness is easy to plan
The crispiness is easy to break
Small pieces are easy to disperse
Prevent at, yet present
Treat at, yet chaos starts
Big tree as one hug
They are born from a small seed
A nine-story high floor
It is erected from a crate of soil
Walking thousands of miles away
But starting with the first step
One who acts fails
One who holds loses
Therefore:
Sage doesn't act
Thereupon he doesn't fail
Doesn't keep
Thereupon he doesn't lose
Things often fail when they are about to be accomplished
Because not as cautious as at first
If the following caution is used as before, the job will not fail
So, the sage avoids ambition

Or precious desire
He wants to teach the uneducated
Help bring people back to the Way
Help things grow naturally
Therefore, one should not interfere with anything.
Chapter 64 – The Book of Ethics

Here are some reasons why you may find balance difficult

1. You are yet to recognize that your life needs balance.

2. There are significant pathways to be balanced you do not know (resources, relationships, self-development, self-maintenance).

- Resources: If the first thing you think of as resources is money, you are sadly missing out on the value in your life. Resources are values that can be traded or substances you require for day-to-day operations.

- Relationships: This is not secluded to a romantic or emotional affiliation. It is how you interact with others, including non-human (plants, animals). As one who is spiritually enlightened, your relationship with the Way is in this category. In addition, as one who seeks to understand themselves, a relationship with yourself is significant.

- Self-development: You must invest in making yourself better. Successful individuals make a constant sacrifice for their skills and upgrade. Whatever form of learning that reshapes you is categorized here. If you do not invest in yourself, you cannot be your greatest motivation, and it will be difficult to fall back on yourself.

- Self-maintenance: This is grooming and taking care of yourself; food, shelter, water, clothing, etc. It is ensuring your biological needs are met

3. You are ignorant of the problems caused by an imbalance.

4. You have not looked out for a means to get balance.

Here are practices that you should engage in to achieve balance

1. Purity: The Way teaches that the body must be pure for the spirit. To be balanced, there are certain things that you should abstain from, like lust, greed, dishonesty, ego, unforgiveness, amongst others. As established already, the inner state of your consciousness affects your physical outlook.

2. Meditation: This is the process of attaining stillness. It is crucial in creating a mental equilibrium and boosting attention. Meditation enables the person the chance to know the Tao directly.

3. Breathing: It is the most straightforward form of ch'i. The breathing exercises carried out by Taoists are numerous and known as Qui Gong.

4. Energy flow: Ch'i is the flow of life energy. It can be increased, controlled, and harmonized by different meditations, exercises, and acupuncture techniques.

5. Martial arts: Tai Chi exercises are also used in achieving balance.

6. Diet: Some food choices should be avoided in Classical Taoism, like meat, beans, alcohol, and grains.

Philosophy of Balance and Tao of Pooh

In the book Tao of Pooh by Benjamin Hoof, he relates Winnie the Pooh by A.A. Milne to Taoism's principles. The book describes a group of wine tasters as great thinkers; Confucius, Buddha, and Lao Tzu.

The character of Winnie the Pooh is likened to the principles of Wu Wei or the concept of effortless living as well as the concept of openness, unburdened. The characters of Owl and Rabbit exaggerate challenges and think to a point where they are confused, the Eeyore is a pessimist who sees everything negatively. Wu-Wei is just like the flow of water in a stream.

Analyzing Pooh's demeanor is a simple character, a humble view of life, and a high problem-solving instinct.

Hence, Pooh is an example of a person living in the Way. There is no greater way to succeed or be ahead in life than to have such essential features. The simplicity in understanding good and bad and the ease in proffering solutions to others is the balance we all desire. Be the balance the world seeks. Some of us do not fully grasp these Wu Wei principles that are linked to the Character of Pooh.

From the character, we see the following principles:

1. *Simplicity, Compassion, and Patience*
   Your greatest treasures in life are the three mentioned above. To be simple in your thoughts and actions, you go back to your source - The Way. By being patient with your friends and foes, you flow with the natural progression of life. Compassion reconciles you with the world's beings.

Lesson to Note: Complications in life occur often but, just like Pooh, do the basics. This did not only help him be balanced but also managed his relationships and actions with the Owl and Rabbit.

2. *Go with the flow*
   A short quote that describes the concept of Wu Wei is "When nothing is done, nothing is left undone." Allow things to take their natural path rather than fight it. No matter the hurdles water faces, it passes through effortlessly, carving a way out for itself naturally. Like water, go through situations without painstakingly creating a path for yourself. If you truly merit it, it will find a way to you.

3. *Let Go*
   Change is inevitable, and death is no respecter of persons. These are the only constants in life. Letting go is tough, but we free ourselves from hurt, pain, and suffering in doing so. Holding on produces double the pain when compared to letting go. By letting things take on their natural path, we don't hold on to anything, regardless of what it may be; a relationship, job opportunity, or what have you.

4. *Harmony*
   The blending of Yin and Yang (femininity and masculinity) brings Harmony; accepting this normalcy and events of things without perceiving it as evil, bad, or dark is balanced.

5. Genuity be true to yourself
   You can only deceive others for a while, but you know the truth. Being true to yourself is wholly embracing everything about you. Only in doing this can you achieve success, take giant strides towards the future, and solicit assistance.

Look but not seeing because of formlessness
Listen but not hearing because of soundlessness
Get it but can't keep it because of being inanimate
Those three things cannot be traced
Because they are one
Above, do not illuminate
Underneath, do not overshadow
It is hard to describe something
When you are far away from it
Then back to nothing
The form of the formless
The shadow of the shadowless
That is called indescribable, non-visualizable
By standing in front, one can't see the head
By following, one can't see the tail
Keep the Way of the past in harmony with the present
Knowing primitiveness is the precept of the Way.
Chapter 14 – The Book of Ethics

Chapter Eight

QIGONG EXERCISE

In previous years, the Qigong exercise was known as Tao You, and Nei Kung translated as leading and guiding. The name describes how the exercise movements direct and lead the transportation of Qi/energy through the body, while Nei Kung translates as internal work/exercise. The dance was a basic foundation of ancient times, so the qigong most likely originated from it. They were initially dance movements created to strengthen dancers and ward off physical and mental diseases, which evolved into exercises and were practiced to maintain health and heal ailments. These practices are massages, breathing, movement, and static exercises for health and long life. The significant insight they passed on is that the flow of life resides in everyone, and by developing it daily, all will attain health and longevity. It is created to assist you in preserving your Jing, transform your Shen, and empower your Qi energy. Qigong is a healing practice that involves breathing, movement, and meditation. Qi is translated as life force while Gong is mastery. It is roughly interpreted as a master of one's energy.

Be open to humiliation
What does "be open to humiliation" mean?
Accept bad luck like its human destiny
Reception is not important
Do not worry about loss or gain
This is called "be open to humiliation"
What does "accept bad luck like it is human destiny" mean?
Bad luck comes from one's body
If not, where does that bad fortune come from?
Be precious to one's body
As people believe one's body is everything
Love this world like one's body
Then one can fulfill everything.
Chapter 13 – The Book of Ethics

The Qigong exercise is a set of repeated movements that are easy to learn, and fun to engage in. Its unique practices possess both Yin, being it, and Yang; doing its traits. Therefore, the Qigong Yin exercises are reflected by calm stretches, breathing techniques, and visualization whereas, the Qigong Yang exercises are reflected by aerobics or in a unique manner. This practice is used largely in China for cancer patients.

The practice of Qigong is supposed to generate energy and vitality of nature into an individual's body to boost mental, spiritual, and physical health. Poor physical health is caused by trapped energy in all body sections based on Traditional Chinese Medicine. The qigong practice has a huge belief in boosting an individual's health by allowing energy to flow through the body. Its purpose is to promote the movement of Qi in the body by making specific gates open while energy sources are stretched and twisted. Relaxing and taking deep breaths are significant to Qigong exercises and necessities for the free flow of energy (Qi).

It invigorates and rejuvenates the body within minutes of engagement and strengthens its various systems (digestive, respiratory, skeletal, cardiovascular, etc.). The Qigong assists in giving treatments for chronic and acute illnesses that are common for exercise, physical and mental healing, relaxation, including other purposes like enlightenment and fighting. There is no preference in age or physique.

In the Qigong practice, some movements are calm and others engaging, extensive, and subtle too. These movements vary from each other and possess unique changes on the body and mind. Naturally, as an individual deepens their Qigong practices, a greater understanding of the movements and its purposes will be gained making the practice fun and desirable.

With consistent practice, Qigong will exhibit a great influence on the mind, spirit, and body. The advantages of this exercise include improved wholeness in health and well-being, decreased stress level, and a balanced and positive mindset on the possibilities of life.

In conclusion, the practice of Qigong can be a discipline, in addition to Tai Chi practices or meditation.

Benefits of Qigong Exercise
The importance of Qigong has been established to have numerous benefits in different areas.

- It harmonizes, strengthens, and has a therapeutic effect on the internal organs and body systems.
- It boosts the production and flow of energy in the body.
- It has a calming and soothing effect on the mental and emotional state.
- It stretches and opens the joints and muscles while releasing muscular tension.
- It completely rejuvenates and nourishes the body by boosting the flow of blood and energy.
- It aids sound sleep, which is a product of relaxation and energization.

Based on Chinese Medicine, the Qi is related to the internal organs of the body. It flows amidst the body extremities like the feet and hands. Hence, when you stretch your upper and lower extremities in defined motions, you will enhance the wellness of the internal organs. Breathing in Qigong is key. The breaths are to be calm, slow, and deeply taken from the diaphragm. The benefit of this breathing method is its calming and soothing influence on the mental state, which effectively suppresses the influence of worry and stress. When you are stressed, engage in some minutes of Qigong, and you will be amazed by the level of relief you experience.

The benefits discussed above are just several positive impacts you will attain at the initial stage of your practice. The more you heighten your commitment and get accustomed to Qigong exercises, the easier it is for you to state the impacts noticed on your body.

Fundamentals Of Qigong Exercises

- *Concentration*
  This begins and yields from the awareness of Qi energy, its breathing formats, and Qigong practices. It involves paying attention and letting go simultaneously. To focus is to expand your awareness by deep relaxation. Here, you will be capable of creating a mind-frame that is sufficient to contain your whole mental, physical, and spiritual abilities and be attentive to create room for worry, distraction, and daily challenges to pass by. The inward focus that enlarges outwardly to be one with you and the universe symbolizes yin/yang.

- *Breathing*
  Lao described the breathing techniques in the sixth century as a means to generate Qi. The two types of breathing are:

The Breath of Buddha: when you breathe in, enlarge your abdomen and fill it with air; to exhale, squeeze your core, expel air from the lung base and push it out until your stomach and chest are relieved from the air. When you inhale and exhale, be imaginative, invite your energy to flow through your body channels freely by using your mind. It should flow with you. Try breathing in for eight counts and out for sixteen counts.

The Breath of Taoist: this technique is opposite from Buddha's. You squeeze your abdomen when breathing in and calm the lungs and torso when you exhale.

As you go through the practices below, do not forget Qigong is to aid awareness.

Warm-Up Practices (1—18 min.)

Qigong Exercise 1: Subtle sway
a. For five minutes, move your arms from shoulders in a calm, swinging manner. This movement originates from your waist: twist from your waist like your trunk is a cloth you are squeezing. It gives massage to the internal organs with maximum benefits. Don't twist from your knees.
b. To begin, move your arms sideways across your trunk and then forward.
c. Allow your knees to bend slightly, and your hips sway. Clear your mind. Pay attention to free up unnecessary and unconscious stress. Weeks later, your focus should be on swinging the arms and Qi movement.

This exercise gives you an insight into being mindful.

Qigong practice 2: Bounce
For starters, try this for about 4 minutes.

a. Keep parallel feet and shoulders apart; like a wet noodle, hang your arms at the sides and bounce with your knees free. Let them feel neutral and empty. While bouncing, your arms in zero position are to get a jiggling influence.

b. Natural shoulders; do not pull or drag them forward. Use the zero position on the general body to get a feel of deep calmness; internal organs and skin should hang. It fosters consciousness of inner tension to enable you to expel it.
The combination of both exercises massages and tones the organ system gently, which aids longevity.

Awareness Practices

Qigong practice 3: Accordion
Here, you experience Qi by using your hands like a bicycle pump/accordion bellow.

a. Your eyes should be closed halfway. Free your mind and focus on your palms.

b. Make your breath slow, simple, and with ease. You are creating a slight trance.

c. Put your hands together, palms touching, and fingers pointing upward. The Laolong (palm chakra) in the center should connect because they are locations where you can feel the Qi.

d. Move your hands slowly, to keep chakras together. At about 30cm distance, move them slowly together with minimal effort.

e. Reduce the air between them like an accordion.

f. Experience a tingling sensation that may be warm at times at the Laolong points.

g. Move your hands slowly, front and back; go through it again in various directions.

This procedure grows Qi, consciousness and enlightens you. Feeling the Qi energy for the first time transforms your mindset.

Qigong Practice 4: Make the point
Your index finger is an excellent way of channeling Qi energy; right-handed people use their right index fingers while left-handed people use their left index fingers. Point at the palm of the other hand, which is perpendicular to the floor, with the fingers pointing upwards.

Using your index finger as a paintbrush, swab to and from across the palm.

Start with your fingertip about 20cm from your palm; move it near and far slowly, swabbing all through.

You may feel a tickly, cooling, and warm sensation.

Qigong Practice 5: Extend Qi
To gather and generate Qi, engage this exercise with half-closed eyes. Qi practices are powerful while at home, have a teacher supervise you, so your eyes don't leak out.

a. Engage with open eyes for stagnant Qi; breath in fast via nostrils with open or half-closed eyes when breathing out.

b. Channel your intention when you sense Qi; this is the mind/spirit aspect so, use your mind to transport your Qi outwards, enlarging your area of comfort. You can pull out Qi as you exhale and hold it as you breathe in.

c. Move the Qi 1 inch from your body; with an increase of 6 inches, take it outward, push for 3 feet, locate the point you are comfortable with and return it close to your body.

These practices make you relate with your Qi. Increasing the distance at which you can feel Qi from your body enlarges your comfort and the world around you. You will experience less fear/deeper abilities. Bringing your Qi to the skin area makes you extra calm, in tune, and self-confident. By learning to increase/reduce Qi, you become healthier, energized, and harmonized within and without.

Qigong Practice 6: Pamper Qi
This practice is tricky, as it moves Qi along two uniquely connecting channels; Du Mai and Ren Mai.

a. Push Qi down; while your hands push down, your spine and head are straight. As the Qi flows up, your hands rise, elbow bend, palms parallel to the floor, hunch shoulders. Repeat about seven times, breathing in as hands go up and out as they come down.

b. When you are comfortable; you can combine this practice with a slow, deliberate walk forward; left knee bent and raised in an overly stepping mode. As the knee comes up, hands go down, back and spine straighten; as footsteps down, hands come up and back hunches. Maintain a breath pattern, gentle and slow feet movement. Breath in as hands raise and out slowly as you straighten the back.

Qigong Practices 7: Blend Qi
This assists you in being conscious of the numerous reverberations of Qi and how to blend them in harmony.

a. With a shoulder apart distance, stand with your feet, slightly bent knees, let your hand hang at the sides.

b. Move your weight to the balls of your feet slightly. Be conscious of the front body region. Focus on the channels that move along the front of legs and trunk, arms, and face.

c. A minute after, transfer the weight to your heels. Be conscious of the back of your body, head, arms, spine, and legs. This position can be held for 5 minutes or more and carried out for both sides of the body.

d. Be conscious of cach part of the body at instances e.g., the side of your head, arm, trunk, leg side, ankle, etc., the exercise becomes meditative this way.

e. Move to a more Nei Dan routine; repeat the first three procedures, without visual movement detection, with your mind, move your weight front and back, perceive your Qi, then try to feel it flow along your front and back together.

Upgraded Qigong Breathing Technique
Through breathing, the Qi energy can be channeled across the body. They can stimulate or relax based on how they are used. Engage this routine (Buddha and Taoist breathing).

- Sit on the ground with crossed legs in lotus or cross. This helps Qi energy refrain from being static at the lower body.

- Breath in at counts 4-8 based on preference. For Buddha, enlarge your abdomen, fill it from the base while for Taoists, breath in and reduce your abdomen, breath out, allow your abdomen to relax.

- Fix your attention on your nose while you inhale. Lead your energy from nose to Dantian (except women on period; on their solar plexus rather) under the navel.

- Breath out to 8-16 count, shift Qi to your torso, pelvic, and tailbone.

- Breath in, shift Qi to the back at the shoulder region

- Breath out, shift Qi to the back at head and nose

Consistency and patience will help you feel the Qi. Increase the rate and finish one cycle in one breath in and out. On breathing in, Qi moves energy from nose to tailbone while breathing out moves from tail to nose.

CONCLUSION

The imbalance caused by the world today proves that humans are in dire need of harmony and balance. The Way is a path that gives insight into spiritual enlightenment, inner peace, balance, harmony, yin and yang principles. Amazingly, it is not restricted to a group of persons or a certain region. All people and nations can practice the Way. It doesn't seek its own glory but rather focuses on achieving peace in this chaotic world of ours. The foundation and principles of the Way are easy to understand and attainable.

Meditation, satisfaction, inner peace, emptiness, and tolerance are the practices one should abide by to connect to mother nature (Earth). As humans, the body, soul, and spirit need harmony. Many of us do not even know that we need the various compositions of our nature to be in perfect sync with each other. Hence the spiritual gap created can only be bridged when we subject ourselves to and are willing to get spiritual enlightenment.

In ancient times, a story was told of a man who had a strange physique that made him stand out from the others. He was sought for within the palace because of the high level of wisdom he expressed. This was all due to his ability to cultivate and maintain his state of consciousness. He was at such peace with himself, balanced from accepting yin and yang, which produced Qi energy enabling him to freely flow with nature and channel its generated Qi to the surroundings and yield outstanding physical attributes. That man was the envy of others who were seemingly normal in physique. He also taught according to the Way - balance is accepting yourself with your perfections and imperfections. It is the beauty of Oneness, yin, and is the beauty of Oneness, Yin and Yang. We cannot all be the same. Life is unique, and our individuality makes it so.

> *A sage does not have a heart of his own*
> *He gets the heart of the world as his heart*
> *One is good to good people*
> *One is also good to those who are not good*
> *Because the essence of Virtue is being good*
> *One believes those who believe*
> *One also believes those who do not believe*
> *Because the essence of Virtue is believing*
> *Sage in the world is carefree*
> *He's in harmony with everyone*
> *So people look and listen*
> *But sage sees them as children.*
> *Chapter 49 - The Book of Ethics*

Diseases, illnesses, issues such as stress, trauma, depression, anxiety, hypertension, panic disorders, bullying, depression, attention disorders, personality disorders, and many stranger medical problems we face today are solely due to our physical, emotional, and mental imbalance. Most of us consume everything the world presents to us hook, line, and sinker, leaving no space for ourselves; instead, we are completely full and probably overflowing with garbage. Does this sound bad? Discouraging? Yes, but do not be distressed. Where there is a will, there is always a way. It is up to you to make a decision, stick to it, be disciplined, take action, and yield results. To be genuinely free, empty, and harmonious, you must work it out.

The Way is the means to escape from the prison the world has put us in because, truthfully, we cannot escape from its violence/chaos. We can only control our response to it. Does the Way teach avoiding situations and circumstances? Does it teach running away from problems? Does it teach one not to confront truth and reality? No, instead, it seeks for you to face your challenges, listen to yourself and thoughts, forget about the past, stop playing the blame/victim card or try to be a perfectionist. Preserve your inner peace by going through the steps mentioned in part 2.

Meditation is a state of stillness that allows you to achieve inner peace and consciousness. Nevertheless, do not forget the first step to spiritual enlightenment is improving your body. The spirit and soul cannot be balanced without a healthy body. The body contains our wills, emotions, insights, etc. When the body is weak, there is little to nothing that can be achieved. The physical (manifesting desire) body, mental (creating the concept) body, and emotional (desiring the concept) body make up the human. The mental manages the emotional, and the emotional controls the physical body.

Accepting ourselves is otherwise known as Self-realization. It is consciously realizing and understanding who we truly are and connecting our personality with the Spirit. Compared to others, individuals who have reached this state are more at peace with themselves and free from the monkey's trap. The monkey's trap is a state when an individual keeps desiring, thinking, and stimulating more to attain satisfaction and happiness. It is a rat race that draws you away from nature, interrupts the flow of the Way, and is the greatest hindrance to self-realization.

The primary purpose of the Taoist concept is humans being at peace with nature and allowing Nature to take its course, that is, handling things, flowing freely.

A story of such goes thus; There was a man who was scared of his shadow and lived in fear of the sound of his footsteps. As he walked alone on a certain day, he panicked and made an effort to run at high speed. However, the faster he ran, the faster his shadow and footsteps caught up with him and made him run the more until he eventually slumped from exhaustion and kicked the bucket.

If he had taken a moment and had only sat at the feet of a tree under its shade, he would not have seen his shadow or heard his footsteps for a while.

Another story is expressed: Once upon a time, a lord wished for a new horse and asked his advisor where he might get a good horse. His advisor pondered for a while and announced that he had a long-time friend who was a professional in the characters of horses and that he would pass messages across to him to get his best horse delivered. Later, a parcel was received from his friend in the country stating that he would be sending a black stallion as a gift to the lord. However, when the horse arrived, it was discovered to be a mare with brown color.

The lord thundered in annoyance, "you said your friend was a professional! Yet, he cannot identify the color or gender of his own horses!"

With a sigh of admiration, the advisor thought aloud, saying, "Alas, has he indeed come this far? A sight so keen that he now cannot perceive things from their outward traits, only the inner virtue matters to him."

These stories have given us a vivid picture with which we can easily connect and understand The Way. It is a simple way of life. The way fosters beauty in all things and satisfaction with everything.

A quality life is attained by balance and harmony. Balance is an all-round thing, it is a combination of emotional, mental, and physical wellbeing. Balance yields a life, ideology, mindset, and a character of positivity. It fosters healthy relationships, a peaceful environment, and a well-developed nation. Harmony works hand-in-hand with balance. Harmony brings all things together, good and bad, to achieve one voice that submits to your inner state. When one aspect of your life loses its balance, it is normal for other aspects of your life to do so too.

A boss once narrated his experience with his employees, particularly the officers, that the stress from work resulted in physical challenges like diabetes, insomnia, high blood sugar, and heart conditions. It is a fact that long periods of stress manifest in depression. Some of the employees were retired athletes, men and women in their mid-forties and early fifties who were expected to be sound physically and mentally due to their previous lifestyle. However, the stress from work had a significant impact on generating and increasing health challenges. The effect of this stress led to a reduction in job satisfaction, frequent sick leave, and prolonged moments from work. In addition to this, there were more complaints and grumbling.

He realized that the problem was that his staff did not understand how they ought to shut off the stress or put a hold on their alertness. It led to the initiation of health challenges related to stress. Their minds were occupied by work; they discuss work away from the office, in their homes, leisure time, etc. They fail to understand that the more you discuss your stressors, the more it takes a toll and stresses you all the more keeping you unbalanced and in chaos with yourself.

By using The Way, this boss took it upon himself to make them conscious of what great future they could achieve if they learned to manage their stressors, alertness, and emotions. The 'Shut the Door on Work' concept was birthed by him to help them leave work at work. A quality life is only achieved when your life is balanced, meaning you have to spend quality time with your family, close friends, have fun doing outdoor activities you love rather than letting work go home with you when you leave work. You cheat yourself and your loved ones from having your company and doing the things that matter.

Discover means to fill your life with positivity; hobbies, fun games, interactive sessions, and activities with family and friends. Take out time alone to unwind and recharge weekly away from the workplace. A mixture of exercise (Qigong exercises, breathing techniques, Tai Chi, mediation), healthy eating, and lifestyle would do great, as discussed in chapter 1 on the importance of the body. Find ways to fill your life with positive activities, fun hobbies, quality time with family and friends, and plenty of personal time to refresh and renew each week when you are away from work. Add to this balance mix exercise, even just walking, and healthy eating.

Furthermore, change how you think about not only work but other areas of your life. The changes, balance, peace, and harmony you want to see will take time, effort, consistency, and practice. Do not relent until practice becomes your way of life.

Act without moving
Do without getting your hands embedded
Taste the tasteless
Increase the small
Make extra the few
Plan the hard work while still easy
Plan the big work while small or not yet present
Hard work in the world
It surely starts from easy
Big work in the world
Surely starts from small
Sages are not doing the big
So, they accomplish the big

Few believe in empty promises
They despise things and face difficulty
Sage considers everything difficult
Therefore, no trouble.
Chapter 63 - The Book of Ethic

NOTES

Part I – The Body

1. What is creationism? - Meaning - Examples- Definition. https://whatdoesmean.net/what-is-creationism/
2. Definition of creationism - What it is, Meaning and.... https://en1.wvpt4learning.org/creacionismo-3788
3. What is creationism? - Meaning - Examples- Definition. https://whatdoesmean.net/what-is-creationism/
4. When your worst enemy is yourself. https://en.psychology instructor.com/when-your-worst-enemy-is-yourself/
5. When Your Worst Enemy Is You - Exploring your mind. https://exploringyourmind.com/when-your-worst-enemy -is-you/
6. When Your Worst Enemy Is Yourself | dayspad.com. https://dayspad.com/when-your-worst-enemy-is-yourself/
7. Gut Brain Connection - The Key to Wellbeing - Jo Spies. https://www.jospies.com.au/blog/gut-brain connection/
8. Best 5 Tips To Achieve Inner Peace. | by The Sky Hustle.... https://theskyhustle.medium.com/best-5-tips-to-achieve-inner-peace-6225d4f3c9cc

Part II – The Spirit

1. Lao Tzu (c.605 BC–c.531 BC) - *Tao Te Ching: The Book of*....https://www.poetryintranslation.com/PITBR/Chinese/TaoTeChing.php
2. Lao Tzu, *The Book of Ethics*, Translated by Tham Trong Ma, 2021.
3. Lão Tử, *Sách Đạo Đức*, Translated by Ma Trọng Thẩm, 2021.
4. Healing Through Nature - Chopra. https://chopra.com/articles/healing-through-nature
5. Philosophy Week 2.docx - *Introduction to the Philosophy of*....https://www.coursehero.com/file/110056520/Philosophy-Week-2docx/
6. Why Mindfulness Is Your Key to Emotional Intelligence | by....https://medium.com/@ttisuccessinsights/why-mindfulness-is-your-key-to-emotional-intelligence-ca584dbf7eb3
7. Water Meditation: Washing Away the Stress [How-To Guide....https://unifycosmos.com/water-meditation-guide/
8. The American president Theodore Roosevelt once said.... https://forallanswers.com/the-american-president-theodore-roosevelt-once-said-comparison-is-the-thief-of-joy-teroa-discusses-how-constant-comparisons-to-her/
9. Healing Through Nature - Chopra. https://chopra.com/articles/healing-through-nature
10. How to find inner peace: 10 things you can start doing.... https://hackspirit.com/how-to-discover-your-inner-peace-in-4-simple-steps/
11. How to Stay Happy During Social Distancing. https://letsreachsuccess.com/happy-during-social-distancing/
12. 7 Ways You Can Be Healthier At Home - The Spirited Puddle....https://www.spiritedpuddlejumper.com/7-ways-you-can-be-healthier-at-home/

13. Happiness: 5 Mistakes You May Be Making. https://letsreachsuccess.com/2014/05/23/happiness-doing-it-wrong/

Part III - The Harmony Of Body And Spirit
1. A Full Disclosure Of The Mysterious Taoist Diet- Natural Healing Dao https://naturalhealingdao.com/a-full-disclosure-of-the-mysterious-taoist-diet
2. Try the Taoist Standing Exercise to Improve Body Alignment and Digestion! https://bodyecology.com/articles/taoist-standing-exercise-php/
3. Secrets of Taoism Longevity and Living a Long Healthy Lifehttps://personaltao.com/tapism/secrets-of-taoism-longevity-and-lifestyle/
4. What are Dantian? The Energy Centers of Chinese Medicine https://www.healthline.com/health/Dantian
5. BBC-Religions-Taoism: Physical practices https://www BBC.co.uk/religion/religions/taoism/practices/physical.shtml
6. Daoist Harmony as a Chinese Philosophy and Psychology https://www.amacad.org/publication/envisioning-daoist-body-economy-cosmic-power
7. https://www.britannica.com/topic/Daoism
8. https://www.holdenqigong.com/history-of-qigong/
9. https://iep.utm.edu/daoism/
10. https://www.google.com/url?sa=t&source=web&rct=j&url=https://philosophynow.org/issues/27/Death_in_Classical_Daoist_Thought&ved=2ahUKEwiRrJ6ttPDzAhVDB2MBHfXjDnEQFnoECCsQAQ&usg=AOvVaw2KUNJqSEnoIq_VYR-pMlOJ

11. https://www.google.com/url?sa=t&source=web&rct=
j&url=https://classroom.synonym.com/what-do-taoists-believe
-about-the-afterlife-12086979.html&ved=2ahUKEwiRrJ6ttPDz
AhVDB2MBHfXjDnEQFnoECDEQAQ&usg=AOvVaw3Beo
2dLC_XfeMv0IqmIOfX

12. https://m.youtube.com/results?sp=mAEA&search_
query=The+psychology+of+harmonization

www.ingramcontent.com/pod-product-compliance
Lightning Source LLC
Chambersburg PA
CBHW061137220326
41599CB00025B/4266